The Sirtfood Diet

How to Lose Weight Easily in 21 Days: Reduce Your Waistline, Burn Fat and Get Toned

MONICA HAWKINS

PUBLISHED BY: Green Book Publishing LTD

58 Warwick Road

London W5 5PX

First Print 2021

are periodically made to this book as and when needed. Where appropriate and/or necessary, you must consult a professional (including but not limited to your doctor, attorney, financial advisor or such other professional advisor) before using any of the suggested remedies, techniques, or information in this book.

Upon using the contents and information contained in this book, you agree to hold harmless the Author from and against any damages, costs, and expenses, including any legal fees potentially resulting from the application of any of the information provided by this book. This disclaimer applies to any loss, damages or injury caused by the use and application, whether directly or indirectly, of any advice or information presented, whether for breach of contract, tort, negligence, personal injury, criminal intent, or under any other cause of action.

You agree to accept all risks of using the information presented inside this book.

You agree that by continuing to read this book, where appropriate and/or necessary, you shall consult a professional (including but not limited to your doctor, attorney, or financial advisor or such other advisor as needed) before using any of the suggested remedies, techniques, or information in this book.

Table of Contents

Introduction 10

    Benefits... 11

Chapter 1: What is Sirt Diet? 14

    Is It Effective? 15

Chapter 2: Sirtuins 18

Chapter 3: Burning Fat.. 21

    Burn Fat 21

Chapter 4: Increase Muscle Mass 26

    Regulation in the Liver 27

Chapter 5: What Are Sirt Foods? 30

    Arugula...30

    Buckwheat...30

    Capers.. 31

    Celery.. 31

    Chilies... 32

    Cocoa 32

    Coffee.. 33

    Extra Virgin Olive Oil................................ 34

    Garlic 34

    Green Tea 34

Kale 35

Medjool Dates 35

Parsley 36

Red Endive 36

Red Onions 36

Red Wine 37

Soy 37

Strawberries 38

Turmeric 38

Walnuts 38

Chapter 6: How It Works and Why It Works 40

First Phase: First 3 days of the week 40

Second Phase: Maintenance 46

Chapter 7: How to Build Your Perfect Diet 48

The Perfect Body Diet 48

What's Your Perfect Weight? 48

What to Eat: Perfect Carbs, Fats, and Proteins 49

Meal Setting 51

The Perfect Body Exercise Program 51

Maintain and Commit Yourself 52

Chapter 8: Maintenance 54

Chapter 9: Easy to Make Recipes – Breakfast Recipes 57

Soy Berry Smoothie 57

Paleolicious Smoothie Bowl 57

Banana-Peanut Butter 'n Greens Smoothie 58

Fruity Tofu Smoothie..59

Green Vegetable Smoothie..60

Creamy Oats, Greens & Blueberry Smoothie 61

Chapter 10: East to Make Recipes – Lunch Bites 62

Potato Bites 62

Salmon and Quinoa Salad..62

Avocado and Salmon Salad Buffet....................................64

Cucumber Salad with Lime and Coriander 65

Salad with salmon and caramelized chicory.....................66

Shrimp, Tomato and Dates Salad 68

Chapter 11: Easy to Make Recipes – Main Meals 69

Curry Chicken with Pumpkin Spaghetti 69

French Style Chicken Thighs 70

Roast Beef with Grilled Vegetables....................................71

Casserole with Spinach and Eggplant................................73

Vegetarian Paleo Ratatouille: 74

Vegan Thai Green Curry 75

Chapter 12: Easy to Make Recipes – Dessert 78

Raw vegan coffee cashew cream cake................................78

Raw vegan chocolate cashew truffles................................79

Raw vegan double almond raw chocolate tart.....................79

Raw vegan "peanut" butter truffles 81

Frozen raw blackberry cake 82

Raw Vegan Chocolate Hazelnuts Truffles 83

Chapter 13: Easy to Make Recipes – Snack 85

Fruity Granola Bars 85

Cardamom Granola Bars 86

Coconut Brownie Bites 87

Tortilla Chips and Fresh Salsa 88

Garlic Baked Kale Chips 90

Cauliflower Nachos...91

Chapter 14: Celebrities Who Are Funs of the Sirtfood Diet 93

Chapter 15: Building a Diet That Works 97

Hitting Your Quota... 98

The Power of Synergy 98

The Power of Protein 100

Eat Early 100

Chapter 16: Sirt Foods...102

Beyond Antioxidants 102

What Doesn't Kill You Makes You Stronger? 103

Enter Polyphenols 104

Chapter 17: Success Stories of Sirt Diet 107

Lorraine Pascale and the Sirtfood diet......................107

David Haye and the Sirtfood diet:.............................108

Jodie Kidd and the Sirt food diet: 109

James Haskell and the Sirt food diet: 110

Sir Ben Ainslie and the Sirt food diet: 111

Adele and the Sirt food diet: 112

Chapter 18: Your 3 Weeks Meal Plan 114

Chapter 19: Sirtfood Diet Theory 121

Evidence 124

Blue Zones 127

Chapter 20: Hacking the Skinny Gene........................... 129

Taking Foods in the Plan That Are Nutritious 129

Diet to Activate Sirtuins and Promote Health..................... 130

Pros and Cons of Sirt food Diet................................. 131

Chapter 21: Exercises and Daily Commitments 134

Eliminate Excess Fat... 135

Tone the Lean Mass 136

Targeted Exercises 138

Various Exercises 138

Chapter 22: 5 Truths in Sirtfood Diet........................... 142

Conclusion 145

FAQ... 149

Is it OK to Exercise During Phase 1 of the Program?........... 149

What's the Purpose of Following This Diet if I'm Already Slim?
.... 149

Is the Sirtfood Diet Right For Me if I'm Obese? 150

I Managed to Reach the Weight I Want, and I Simply Don't Want to Lose Any More Weight. Do I have to Stop Eating sirt Foods?..150

I've Just Finished Phase 2. Do I Need to Stop Drinking the Green Juice? 151

Is it OK to Follow This Diet if I Take Medication? 151

Can Children Try This Diet?... 151

Introduction

Experiencing difficulty in searching for a complete and accurate guide to weight reduction, search no more. This book will take you to a safer and sexier body with the best and most positive acts. Unlike other devices that focus only on a single part of the diet, this book will feature all you need to know about weight reduction.

Fasting-based diets have become very popular over the past few years. Studies show that by fasting - that is, with moderate daily calorie restriction or by practicing a more radical, but less frequent, intermittent fast - you can expect to lose about 3 kg in a month and substantially reduce the risk of contracting certain diseases.

According to the Sirt food Diet, it is. A skinny gene that, if appropriately activated, allows you to lose weight and gain health altogether. The singer Adele has lost 30 kilos in a year thanks to this philosophy: a program of two medical nutritionists, Aidan Goggins and Glen Matten, which is based on the introduction of some Sirt foods in our diet.

These are particularly nutrient-rich foods capable of activating the same skinny genes stimulated by fasting. These genes are called sirtuins and considered to be super regulators of metabolism to influence our ability to burn fat.

By eating a diet rich in Sirt foods, participants are claimed to lose weight, gain muscle, look and feel better and perhaps even live a longer and healthier life.

It is a diet that is hailed as the next 5:2 and has a whole host of celebrities promoting this. The Sirt Food Diet is not just about weight loss but also about improving overall health and well-being, longevity, and resistance to disease.

So, what are the magic sirtfoods? The ten most frequently used include green tea, dark chocolate (that is at least 85% cocoa), apples, blueberries, capers, citrus fruits, parsley, red wine, turmeric, kale. Sirtfood diet is a two-phase approach; the initial phase in lasts one week and involves a three-day reduction of calories to 1000kcal consuming three sirt food green juices & one meal per day.

Benefits

No doubt, eating Sirt foods is right for you as they are full of healthy plant compounds and rich in nutrients.

Studies have also shown that most of the foods recommended on this diet have several health benefits.

For instance, consuming a moderate amount of dark chocolate rich in cocoa content helps to fight inflammation in the body and lowers your risk of heart diseases.

Consuming green tea helps to lower blood pressure as well as reduce your risk of diabetes and stroke.

Turmeric has also been proven to have anti-inflammatory properties beneficial to the body in general while protecting you against inflammation-related diseases.

While studies on the health benefits of this diet are still ongoing, research in cell lines and animals have provided exciting results.

For instance, research showed that increased levels of specific sirtuin protein caused a longer lifespan in mice, worms, and yeast.

Also, during calorie restriction or fasting, the sirtuin protein alerts your body to burn more fat for energy as well as improve your insulin sensitivity. One study in mice showed that increased levels of sirtuin led to the loss of fat in the body.

Other evidence shows that sirtuins help to slow the development of Alzheimer's and heart disease, reduce inflammation, and inhibit tumor development.

Although Sirt foods are not a mainstay of nutrition in most of the western world today, the situation was quite different in the past. They were a fundamental element, and if many have become rare and others have even disappeared, it is definitely possible to reverse the course of this.

Our good news for you is that you don't have to be a top athlete, and not even sporty, to enjoy the same benefits.

We took advantage of everything we learned about Sirt foods thanks to the pilot study by KX and the work done with athletes, and we adapted it to create a diet suitable for anyone who wants to lose weight while improving health.

We've distinguished facts from fiction to show you everything about the Sirt food Diet you need to know. Please continue reading to find out the SIRT diet and whether it is perfect for you.

Chapter 1: What is Sirt Diet?

Sirt Diet has gotten the most loved of big names in Europe and is popular for permitting red wine and chocolate.

Its makers demand that it is anything but a prevailing fashion, yet rather than "sirt foods" are the key to opening fat misfortune and forestalling malady.

In any case, wellbeing specialists caution that this eating routine may not satisfy everyone's expectations and could even be a poorly conceived notion.

Two VIP nutritionists working for a private rec center in the UK built up the Sirt Food Diet.

They publicize the eating regimen as a progressive new eating regimen and wellbeing plan that works by turning on your "thin quality."

This eating regimen depends on investigating on sirtuins (SIRTs), a gathering of seven proteins found in the body that has been appeared to manage an assortment of capacities, including digestion, irritation, and life expectancy.

The eating regimen consolidates sirt foods and calorie limitation, the two of which may trigger the body to create more significant levels of sirtuins.

The Sirt Food Diet book incorporates feast plans and plans to follow, yet there are a lot of other Sirt food Diet formula books accessible.

The eating routine's makers guarantee that following the Sirt Food Diet will prompt fast weight reduction, all while keeping up bulk and shielding you from interminable illness.

When you have finished the eating routine, you are urged to keep including sirt foods and the eating regimen's mark green juice into your normal eating routine.

The Sirt Food Diet depends on look into on sirtuins, a gathering of proteins that direct a few capacities in the body. Certain nourishments called sirt foods might make the body produce a greater amount of these proteins.

Is It Effective?

The creators of the Sirt Food Diet make intense cases, including that the eating regimen can super-charge weight reduction, turn on your "thin quality" and forestall sicknesses.

The issue is there isn't a lot of confirmation to back them.

Up until this point, there's no persuading proof that the Sirt Food Diet has a more helpful impact on weight reduction than some other calorie-limited eating routine.

Furthermore, albeit a considerable lot of these nourishments have restorative properties, there have not been any long-haul human investigations to decide if eating an eating routine rich in sirt foods has any substantial medical advantages.

By and by, the Sirt Food Diet book reports the aftereffects of a pilot study directed by the writers and including 39 members from their wellness focus. In any case, the aftereffects of this examination show up not to have been distributed anyplace else.

For the multi-week, the members followed the eating regimen and practiced every day. Toward the week's end, members lost a normal of 7 pounds (3.2 kg) and kept up or even picked up the bulk.

However, these outcomes are not really amazing. Confining your calorie admission to 1,000 calories and practicing simultaneously will about consistently cause weight reduction.

Notwithstanding, this sort of speedy weight reduction is neither authentic nor durable, and this investigation didn't follow members after the primary week to check whether they restored any of the weight, which is normally the situation.

At the point when your body is vitality denied, it goes through its crisis vitality stores, or glycogen, notwithstanding consuming fat and muscle.

Every atom of glycogen requires 3–4 particles of water to be put away. At the point when your body goes through glycogen, it disposes of this water too. It's known as "water weight."

In the principal seven day stretch of extraordinary calorie limitation, just around 33% of the weight reduction originates from fat, while the other 66% originates from water, muscle, and glycogen.

When your calorie admission expands, your body recharges its glycogen stores, and the weight returns right.

Sadly, this sort of calorie limitation can likewise make your body bring down its metabolic rate, causing you to need significantly fewer calories every day for vitality than previously.

Almost certainly, this eating regimen may assist you with shedding a couple of pounds first and foremost, yet it will probably return when the eating routine is finished.

To the extent of forestalling sickness, three weeks is presumably not long enough to have any quantifiable long-haul sway.

Then again, adding Sirt foods to your normal eating routine over the long haul might just be a smart thought. Be that as it may, all things considered, you should skirt the eating regimen and start doing that now.

Chapter 2: Sirtuins

Sirtuins are a group of proteins that manage cell wellbeing. Sirtuins assume a key job in controlling cell homeostasis.

Protein may seem like dietary protein from beans and meats— yet for this situation, we're discussing proteins that work all through the body's phones in various capacities. Consider proteins the divisions at an organization, everyone concentrating without anyone else explicit capacity while planning with different offices.

Sirtuins are with acetyl bunches by doing what's called deacetylation. Sirtuins' work is by evacuating acetyl gatherings deacetylating organic proteins, for example, histones.

We've just thought about sirtuins, and their essential capacity was found during the 1990s. From that point forward, specialists have rushed to examine them, recognizing their significance while likewise bringing up issues about what else we can find out about them.

Diet displayed a decrease of coronary illness chance related to lower plasma cholesterol and incendiary files in contrast with members on a sound, for the most part, vegan diet.

Nonetheless, additionally, the measure of ingested nourishment has been pulling in light of a legitimate concern for mainstream researchers as a potential modifier of the harmony among wellbeing and infection in a wide range of living species. Specifically, calorie limitation CR has been exhibited to be a rising healthful intercession that animates the counter maturing instruments in the body.

There are seven types of Sirtuins named SIRT1 to SIRT7. Although our understanding of the exact functions of all the Sirtuins is minimal, studies show that activating them can have the following benefits: switching on fat burning and protection from weight gain: Sit-ins do this by increasing the functionality of the mitochondrion which is involved in the production of energy and sparking a change in your metabolism to break down more fat cells and improving memory by protecting neurons from damage. Sirtuins also boost learning skills and memory through the enhancement of synaptic plasticity. The synaptic plasticity refers to the ability of synapses to weaken or strengthen with time due to a decrease or increase in their activity. This is important because memories are represented by different interconnect networks of synapses in the brain, and synaptic plasticity is an important neurochemical foundation of memory and learning.

Slowing down the Ageing Process: sirtuins act as cell guarding enzymes. Thus, they protect the cells and slow down their aging process.

Repairing cells: The sirtuins repair cells damaged by re-activating cell functionality.

Protection against diabetes: this happens through prevention against insulin resistance. Sirtuins do this by controlling blood sugar levels because this diet calls for moderate consumption of carbohydrates. These foods cause increases in blood sugar levels, hence the need to release insulin, and as the blood sugar levels increase greatly, there is a need to produce more insulin. Over time, cells become resistant to insulin; hence, the need to produce more insulin, and this leads to insulin resistance.

Fighting Cancers: The chemicals working as sirtuin activators affect the function of sirtuin in different cells, i.e., by switching it on when in normal cells and shutting it down in cancerous cells. This encourages the death of cancerous cells.

Fighting inflammation: sirtuins have a powerful antioxidant effect that has the power to reduce oxidative stress. This has positive effects on heart health and cardiovascular protection.

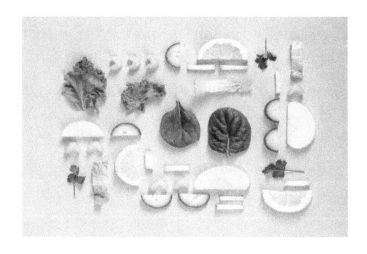

Chapter 3: Burning Fat

The Sirt food Diet was originally developed to help promote health and fight disease, and the impressive weight loss benefits were merely a surprising and happy bonus. As such, this way of eating is deeply rooted in scientific data and medical research.

Following a prescriptive diet that tells you exactly what to eat and when might be useful for a few weeks, but it won't be sustainable. In order to make changes that last a lifetime and that you are whole-heartedly committed to, you must understand why you're making these changes.

Burn Fat

In addition to protecting your muscles, sirt foods encourage your metabolic system to start burning through the fat that is stored in your body, which is one of the reasons for the surprising weight loss potential.

Gaining weight is a complex process for humans that involves multiple hormones sending signals back and forth to your various biological processes. One of these hormones, insulin, I'm sure you're familiar with.

When you consume any calories, your body needs to convert the food into glucose so that it can be used as energy to keep your body functioning. Some foods, such as sugar or refined carbohydrates, for example, convert to sugar in your bloodstream almost instantaneously, causing a spike in blood glucose levels.

Other foods, like complex carbohydrates and proteins, take longer for your body to break down and convert to glucose, so your blood gets a more slow and steady drip of glucose.

If your blood sugar gets too high because you've consumed more sugar than your body needs to operate immediately, it can cause a variety of problems. Headaches, thirst, or fatigue might be experienced in the short-term, but high blood sugar levels can lead to kidney failure, heart disease, or nerve damage if the issue becomes chronic.

Obviously, these symptoms are severe and potentially life-threatening, so your body has a process to detect high blood sugar levels and bring them back down: it releases insulin.

With the help of your liver and cholesterol, insulin pulls sugar out of your bloodstream and tells your cells to take it in instead, and your blood glucose levels drop as your fat cells get a little fuller.

When your blood sugar gets too low, another hormone, glucagon, will be released. Glucagon taps your liver and fat cells in order to release the stored glucose back into your bloodstream.

The main problem with our modern diet is that humans have developed the habit of constant grazing and/or over-eating. This provides a constant flow of glucose, triggering a constant need for insulin. Our blood sugar rarely dips low enough to trigger the production of glucagon, so instead of using our stored energy, we simply add more to the reserves.

Swapping a Standard American Diet (SAD) that causes an instant spike in your blood glucose for a Sirt food Diet, which will create a more slow and steady flow of energy will help to reinstate that natural balance of hormones once again. As an added bonus, studies have shown that activating sirtuins can actually suppress your body's ability to store fat as it increases the propensity to burn it (Picard et al., 2004). Your metabolic system will actually have a chance to use the stored energy.

Aside from sirtfoods being a more balancing form of energy, by activating our sirtuin genes, our cells are being protected and fortified. Each cell has a power center called a mitochondrion, which is responsible for the conversion of glucose into useable energy. This is a lot of work for our cells, and, especially if we are eating more calories than we need and those calories are primarily simple carbohydrates, our mitochondria wear out quickly.

Sirtuins protect our mitochondria, allowing them to process energy more efficiently. In other words, we can burn fat more quickly.

Sirtfoods work on multiple fronts to help our body naturally regulate weight: they reduce the amount of glucose that gets stored as fat, and they increase the speed at which our fat gets used.

As an added bonus, by naturally regulating our metabolism, we can protect ourselves against insulin resistance and type 2 diabetes.

Insulin and glycogen aren't the only hormones to return to a healthy balance on a Sirt food Diet. Leptin is also regulated.

Leptin resistance isn't as commonly understood as insulin resistance, but it plays just as important of a role in the process of weight gain. Leptin is often called the hunger hormone because it's responsible for telling your brain when you have enough fat stored in your body to keep you safe, and when you need to take in more energy.

If you have low body fat, your brain will throw out hunger signals to encourage you to eat more food. Unfortunately, if you have damaged leptin receptors, your brain will also continue to pump out hunger signals, whether you're actually in need of energy or not.

Hunger is very hard to ignore, and if your leptin levels are dysregulated, not only are you going to feel hungry constantly, but your body will also be actively trying to store any energy you consume as fat instead of using it immediately.

When you follow a Sirt food Diet, your leptin levels will naturally balance, and your hunger signals will only start to spark when you truly need more nutrition, not simply when your sugar crash has taken a turn for the worse.

When all the hormones associated with your metabolism are operating and communicating effectively, you will only store as much body fat as necessary for your health. If you're currently overweight, repairing your metabolic system will help you release weight quickly, until you have reached your optimal body composition.

Chapter 4: Increase Muscle Mass

SIRT1, just like other SIRTUINS family, is protein NAD+ dependent deacetylases that are associated with cellular metabolism. All sirtuins, including SIRT1 important for sensing energy status and in protection against metabolic stress. They coordinate cellular response towards Caloric Restriction (CR) in an organism. SIRT1 diverse location and allows cells to easily sense changes in the level of energy anywhere in the mitochondria, nucleus, and cytoplasm. They were associated with metabolic health through DE acetylation of several target proteins such as muscles, Liver, endothelium, heart, and adipose tissue.

SIRT1, SIRT6, and SIRT7 are localized in the nucleus where they take part in the DE acetylation of customers to influence gene expression epigenetically. SIRT2 is located in the cytosol, while SIRT3, SIRT4, and SIRT5 are located in the mitochondria where they regulate metabolic enzyme activities as well as moderate oxidative stress.

SIRT1, as most studies with regards to metabolism, aid in mediating the physiological adaptation to diets. Several studies have shown the impact of sirtuins on Caloric Restriction. Sirtuins deacetylase non-histone proteins that define pathways involved during the metabolic adaptation when there are metabolic restrictions. Caloric Restriction, on the other hand, causes the induction of expression of SIRT1 in humans.

Mutations that lead to loss of function in some sirtuins genes can lead to a reduction in the outputs of caloric restrictions. Therefore, sirtuins have the following metabolic functions:

Regulation in the Liver

The Liver regulates the body glucose homeostasis. During fasting or caloric restriction, glucose level becomes low, resulting in a sudden shift in hepatic metabolism to glycogen breakdown and then to gluconeogenesis to maintain glucose supply as well as ketone body production to mediate the deficit in energy. Also, during caloric restriction or fasting, there is muscle activation and liver oxidation of fatty acids produced during lipolysis in white adipose tissue. For this switch to occur, there are several transcription factors involved to adapt to energy deprivation. SIRT1 intervenes during the metabolic switch to see the energy deficit.

At the initial stage of the fasting that is the post glycogen breakdown phase, there is the production of glucagon by the pancreatic alpha cells to active gluconeogenesis in the Liver through the cyclic amp response element-binding protein (CREB), and CREB regulated transcription coactivator 2 (CRTC2), the coactivator. Is the fasting gets prolonged, the effect is canceled out and is being replaced by SIRT1 mediated CRTC2 deacetylase resulting in targeting of the coactivator for ubiquitin/ proteasome-mediated destruction? SIRT1, on the other hand, initiates the next stage of gluconeogenesis through acetylation and activation of peroxisome proliferator-activated receptor coactivator one alpha, which is the coactivator necessary for fork head box O1. In addition to the ability of SIRT1 to support gluconeogenesis, coactivator one alpha is required during the mitochondrial biogenesis necessary for the Liver to accommodate the reduction in energy status. SIRT1 also activates fatty acid oxidation through deacetylation and activation of the nuclear receptor to increase energy production. SIRT1, when involved in acetylation and repression of glycolytic enzymes such as phosphoglycerate mutate 1, can lead to shutting down of the production of energy through glycolysis. SIRT6, on the other hand, can be served as a co-repressor for hypoxia-inducible Factor 1 Alpha to repress glycolysis. Since SIRT6 can transcriptionally be induced by SIRT1, sirtuins can coordinate the duration of time for each fasting phase.

Aside from glucose homeostasis, the Liver also overtakes in lipid and cholesterol homeostasis during fasting. When there are caloric restrictions, the synthesis of fat and cholesterol in the Liver is turned off, while lipolysis in the white adipose tissue commences. The SIRT1, upon fasting, causes acetylation of steroid regulatory element-binding protein (SREBP) and targets the protein to destroy the ubiquitin-professor system. The result is that fat cholesterol synthesis will repress. During the regulation of cholesterol homeostasis, SIRT1 regulates the oxysterol receptor, thereby assisting the reversal of cholesterol transport from peripheral tissue through up regulation of the oxysterol receptor target gene ATP-binding cassette transporter A1 (ABCA1).

Further modulation of the cholesterol regulatory loop can be achieved via bile acid receptor, that's necessary for the biosynthesis of cholesterol catabolic and bile acid pathways. SIRT6 also participates in the regulation of cholesterol levels by repressing the expression and post-translational cleavage of SREBP1/2, into the active form. Furthermore, in the circadian regulation of metabolism, SIRT1 participates through the regulation of cell circadian clock.

Mitochondrial SIRT3 is crucial in the oxidation of fatty acid in mitochondria. Fasting or caloric restrictions can result in the up-regulation of activities and levels of SIRT3 to aid fatty acid oxidation through deacetylation of long-chain specific acyl-CoA dehydrogenase. SIRT3 can also cause activation of ketogenesis and the urea cycle in the Liver.

SIRT1 also Add it in the metabolic regulation in the muscle and white adipose tissue. Fasting causes an increase in the level of SIRT1, leading to DE acetylation of coactivator one alpha, which in turn causes genes responsible for fat oxidation to get activated. The reduction in energy level also activates AMPK, which will activate the expression of coactivator one alpha. The combined effects of the two processes will give rise to increased mitochondrial biogenesis together with fatty acid oxidation in the muscle.

Chapter 5: What Are Sirt Foods?

Arugula

(also known as rocket, rucola, arugula, and roquette) has a colorful history in American food culture. A pungent green salad leaf with a distinctive peppery taste, it rapidly rose from humble roots to become an emblem of food snobbery in the United States as the source of many peasant dishes in the Mediterranean, thus contributing to the coining of the word arugulance.

Buckwheat

Buckwheat was one of Japan's earliest domesticated crops, and the story goes that when Buddhist monks made long trips into the mountains, they'd just bring a cooking pot and a buckwheat bag for food. Buckwheat is so nutritious that this was all they needed, and it fed them up for weeks. We're big fans of buckwheat too. Firstly, because it is one of a sirtuin activator's best-known sources, called rutin. But also, because it has advantages as a cover crop, improving soil quality and suppressing weed growth, making it a fantastic crop for environmentally sound and sustainable agriculture.

Capers

In case you're not so familiar with capers, we're talking about those salty, dark green, pellet-like things on top of a pizza that you may only have had occasion to see. Yet inevitably, they are one of the most undervalued and overlooked foods out there. Intriguingly, they are the caper bush's flower buds, which grow abundantly in the Mediterranean before being picked and preserved by hand. Studies now reveal that capers possess important antimicrobial, anti-diabetic, anti-inflammatory, immune-modulatory, and antiviral properties, and have a history of medicinal use in the Mediterranean and North African regions. It's hardly shocking when we find that they are filled with nutrients that trigger sirtuin.

Celery

For centuries, celery was around and revered — with leaves still adorning the ashes of the Egyptian pharaoh Tutankhamun who died about 1323 BCE. Early strains were very bitter, and celery was generally considered a medicinal plant, especially for cleansing and detoxification to prevent disease. This is especially interesting given that liver, kidney, and gut health are among the many promising benefits that science is now showing. In the seventeenth century, it was domesticated as a vegetable, and selective breeding reduced its strong bitter flavor in favor of sweeter varieties, thus establishing its place as a traditional salad vegetable—abundantly in the Mediterranean before being picked and preserved by hand.

Chilies

The chili has been an integral part of gastronomic experience worldwide for thousands of years. On one level, it's disconcerting that we'd be so enamored with it. The pungent fire, caused by a substance called capsaicin in chilies, is engineered as a method of plant protection to cause pain and dissuade pests from feasting on it, and we appreciate that. The food and our infatuation with it are almost magical.

Incredibly, one study showed that consuming chilies together even enhances human cooperation. So we know from a health perspective that their seductive fire is wonderful to stimulate our sirtuins so improve our metabolism. The culinary applications of the chili are also endless, making it an easy way to give a hefty Sirt food boost to any dish.

Cocoa

Cocoa was considered a holy food and was usually reserved for the elite and the warriors, served at feasts to gain loyalty and duty.

Unfortunately, there's no count here for the diluted, refined, and highly sweetened milk chocolate we commonly munch. We're talking about chocolate with

85% solids of cocoa to earn its Sirt food badge. But even then, aside from the percentage of cocoa, not every chocolate is created equal. To the acidity to give it a darker color, chocolate is often handled with an alkalizing agent (known as the Dutch process). Sadly, this process diminishes its sirtuin-activating flavones massively, thereby seriously compromising its health-promoting quality. Fortunately, and unlike in many other countries, food labelling regulations in the United States require alkalized cocoa to be declared as such and labelled "alkali processed." We recommend avoiding these products, even if they boast a higher percentage of cocoa, and opting instead for those who have not undergone Dutch processing to reap the real benefits of cocoa.

Coffee

This is why coffee drinkers have low rates of certain cancers and neurodegenerative diseases. As for that ultimate irony, rather than being a toxin, coffee protects our livers and makes them healthier! And on the other hand, to the popular belief that coffee dehydrates the body, it is now well established not to be the case, with coffee (and tea) making a perfect contribution to the fluid intake of regular coffee drinkers.

Extra Virgin Olive Oil

There is now a rich scientific data showing that regular olive oil consumption is highly cardio-protective, as well as playing a role in reducing the risk of major modern-day diseases such as diabetes, certain cancers, and osteoporosis, and associated with increased longevity.

Garlic

One of Nature's wonder foods for thousands of years, with healing and rejuvenating powers. Egyptians feed pyramid workers with garlic to enhance their defenses, avoid various diseases, and improve their performance by their ability to prevent exhaustion. Garlic naturally an antibiotic and antifungal that is often used to help treat ulcers in the stomach.

Green Tea

Many will be acquainted with green tea, the toast of the Orient, and ever more common in the West. As the growing awareness of its health benefits, green tea intake is related to less obesity, heart disease, diabetes, and osteoporosis. The explanation it is believed that green tea is so healthy for us is primarily due to its rich content of a group of powerful plant compounds named catechins, the star of the show is a particular type of sirtuin-activating catechin known as epigallocatechin gallate (EGCG).

We like to think of matcha on the steroids as normal green tea. In contrast to traditional green tea, which is prepared as an infusion, it is a special powdered green tea which is prepared by dissolving directly in water. The upshot of consuming matcha is that it contains dramatically higher levels of the sirtuin-activating compound EGCG than other green tea types.

Kale

We've done the research, filled with suspicions, and we have to admit that we conclude that kale deserves her pleasures (although we still don't recommend the T-shirts!). The reason we're pro-kale is that it boasts bumper amounts of the quercetin and kaempferol sirtuin-activating nutrients, making it a must-include in the Sirt Food Diet and the base of our green Sirt food juice. What's so refreshing about kale is that kale is available everywhere, locally grown, and very affordable, unlike the usual exotic, hard-to-source, and exorbitantly priced so-called super foods.

Medjool Dates

It may come as a surprise to include Medjool dates in a list of foods that stimulate weight loss and promote health — especially when we tell you that Medjool dates contain a staggering 66% sugar. Sugar doesn't have any sirtuin-activating properties at all; rather, it has well-established links to obesity, heart disease, and diabetes

— just the opposite of what we're looking for to achieve. But processed and replenished sugar is very different from sugar carried in a nature-borne vehicle balanced with sirtuin-activating polyphenols: the date Medjool.

Parsley

Taste aside, what makes parsley special is that it is an excellent source of the sirtuin-activating nutrient apigenin, a real boon since it is seldom found in other foods in significant quantities. In our brains, apigenin binds fascinatingly to the benzodiazepine receptors, helping us to relax and help us to sleep. Stack it all up, and it's time we enjoyed parsley not as omnipresent food confetti, but as a food in its own right to reap the wonderful health benefits that it can bring.

Red Endive

Endive is now grown all over the world, including the USA, and earns its Sirt food badge thanks to its impressive sirtuin activator luteolin content. And besides the established sirtuin-activating benefits, luteolin consumption has become a promising approach to therapy to improve sociability in autistic children.

Red Onions

Sirt food status because they're chock-full of the sirtuin-activating compound quercetin — the very compound that the sports science world has recently started actively researching and marketing to improve sports performance.

And why the red ones? Simply because they have the highest content of quercetin, although the standard yellow ones do not lag too far behind and are also a good inclusion.

Red Wine

Naturally, in 2003, the rich content of red wine from a bevy of sirtuin-activating nutrients was uncovered, and the rest, as they say, was made history.

But there is even more to the impressive resume in red wine. Red wine seems to be able to keep away from the common cold, with moderate wine drinkers having an incidence reduction of more than 40 percent. Research now also shows advantages for oral health and cavity protection.

Soy

Researchers first turned on to soy after finding that high soy-consuming countries had significantly lower rates of certain cancers, particularly breast and prostate cancers. This is due to a special group of polyphenols in soybeans known as isoflavones, which may favorably change how estrogens work in the body, including daidzein and formononetin sirtuin-activators. Soy product consumption has also been linked to a reduction in the incidence or severity of a variety of conditions such as cardiovascular disease, symptoms of menopause, and bone loss.

Strawberries

Intriguingly, and inherently low in sugar itself, strawberries have pronounced effects on how the body handles carbohydrates. What researchers have found is that adding strawberries to carbohydrates reduces the demand for insulin, essentially turning the food into a sustained energy releaser. Yet new research also shows that eating strawberries in diabetes care has similar effects on drug therapy.

Turmeric

One factor that prevents turmeric's potency is that its main sirtuin-activating compound, curcumin when we consume it. Research, however, shows that we can overcome this by cooking it in liquid, adding fat, and adding black pepper, all of which absorption increases dramatically.

Walnuts

The emerging research showing walnuts to be a powerful anti-aging food is less well known but equally intriguing. Evidence often refers to their advantages as a brain food with the ability to slow down brain aging and reduce the risk of degenerative brain diseases, as well as reducing the deterioration of physical function with age.

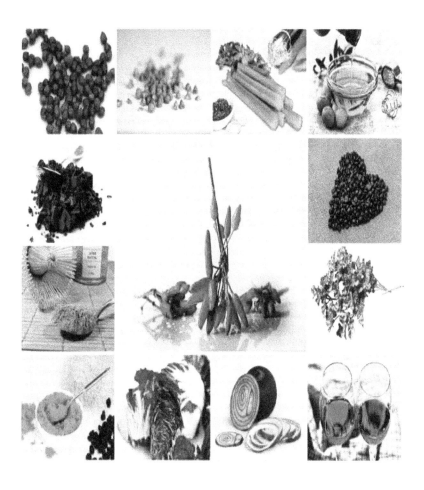

Chapter 6: How It Works and Why It Works

First Phase: First 3 days of the week

Monday: 3 green juices

- Breakfast: water + tea or espresso + a cup of green juice;
- Lunch: green juice
- Snack: a cup of green juice;
- Dinner: Sirt meal
- After dinner: a square of dark chocolate.

Drink the juices at three distinct times of the day (for example, in the morning as soon as you wake up, mid-morning and mid-afternoon) and choose the normal or vegan dish: pan-fried oriental prawns with buckwheat spaghetti or miso and tofu with sesame glaze and sautéed vegetables (vegan dish)

Tuesday: 3 green juices

- Breakfast: water + tea or espresso + a cup of green juice
- Lunch: 1 green juice;
- Snack: 1 green juice
- Dinner: Sirt meal

- After dinner: a square of dark chocolate.

Welcome to day 2 of the Sirt Food Diet. The formula is identical to that of the first day, and the only thing that changes is the solid meal. Today you will also have dark chocolate, and the same goes for tomorrow. This food is so wonderful that we don't need an excuse to eat it.

To earn the title of a "Sirt food", chocolate must be at least 85 percent cocoa. And even among the various types of chocolate with this percentage, not all of them are the same. Often this product is treated with an alkalizing agent (this is the so-called "Dutch process") to reduce its acidity and give it a darker color. Unfortunately, this process greatly reduces the flavonoids activating sirtuins, compromising their health benefits.

On the second day, you will intake 3 green Sirt juices and one solid meal (normal or vegan).

Wednesday: 3 green juices

- Breakfast: water + tea or espresso + a cup of green juice

- Lunch: 2 green juices before dinner;

- Snack: a square of dark chocolate;

- Dinner: Sirt meal

- After dinner: a square of dark chocolate.

You are now on the third day, and even if the format is once again identical to that of days 1 and 2, so the time has come to flavor everything with a fundamental ingredient. For thousands of years, chili has been a fundamental element of the gastronomic experiences of the whole world. This is the last day you will consume three green juices a day; tomorrow, you will switch to two. We, therefore, take this opportunity to browse other drinks that you can have during the Diet.

As for the effects on health, we have already seen that its spiciness is perfect for activating sirtuins and stimulating the metabolism. The applications of chili are endless, and therefore represent an easy way to consume Sirt food regularly.

On the third day, you will intake 3 green Sirt juices and 1 one solid meal (normal or vegan, see below).

Thursday: 2 green juices

- Breakfast: water + tea or espresso + a cup of green juice;
- Lunch: Sirt food;
- Snack: 1 green juice before dinner
- Dinner: Sirt food

The fourth day of the Sirt Food Diet has arrived, and you are halfway through your journey to a leaner and healthier body. The big change from the last three days is that you will only drink two juices instead of three and that you will have two solid meals instead of one. This means that on the fourth day and the upcoming ones, you will have two green juices and 2 solid meals, all delicious and rich in Sirt foods. The inclusion of Medjoul dates in a list of foods that promote weight loss and good health may seem surprising. Especially when you think they contain 66 percent sugar.

On the fourth day, you will intake: 2 green Sirt juices, 2 solid meals (normal or vegan)

Friday: 2 green juices

- Breakfast: water + tea or espresso + a cup of green juice
- Lunch: Sirt food
- Snack: a green juice before dinner;
- Dinner: Sirt food

You have reached the fifth day, and the time has come to add fruits. Due to its high sugar content, fruits have been the subject of bad publicity. This does not apply to berries. Strawberries have a very low sugar content: one tsp per 100 grams. They also have an excellent effect on how the body processes simple sugars.

On the fifth day, you will intake 2 green Sirt juices and 2 solid meals (normal or vegan).

Saturday: 2 green juices

- Breakfast: water + tea or espresso + a cup of green juice
- Lunch: Sirt food
- Snack: a green juice before dinner;

- Dinner: Sirt food

There are no Sirt foods better than olive oil and red wine. Virgin olive oil is obtained from the fruit only by mechanical means, in conditions that do not deteriorate it, so that you can be sure of its quality and polyphenol content. "Extra virgin" oil is that of the first pressing ("virgin" is the result of the second) and therefore has more flavor and better quality: this is what we strongly recommend you to use when cooking.

No Sirt menu would be complete without red wine, one of the cornerstones of the Diet. It contains the activators of resveratrol and piceatannol sirtuins, which probably explain the longevity and slenderness associated with the traditional French way of life, and which are at the origin of the enthusiasm unleashed by Sirt foods.

On the sixth day, you will assume 2 green Sirt juices and 2 solid meals (normal or vegan).

Drink the juices at different times of the day (for example, the first in the morning as soon as you wake up or in the middle of the morning, the second in the middle of the afternoon) and choose the normal or vegan dishes: Super Sirt salad and grilled beef fillet with red wine sauce, onion rings, curly garlic kale and roasted potatoes with aromatic herbs or

Super lentil Sirt salad (vegan dish) and mole sauce of red beans with roasted potato (vegan dish).

Sunday: 2 green juices

- Breakfast: a bowl of Sirt Muesli + a cup of green juice

- Lunch: Sirt food

- Snack: a cup of green juice;

- Dinner: Sirt food

The seventh day is the last of phase 1 of the Diet. Instead of considering it as an end, see it as a beginning, because you are about to embark on a new life, in which Sirt foods will play a central role in your nutrition. Today's menu is a perfect example of how easy it is to integrate them in abundance into your Daily Diet. Just take your favorite dishes, and, with a pinch of creativity, you will turn them into a Sirt banquet.

On the seventh day, you will assume 2 green Sirt juices; 2 solid meals (normal or vegan).

Drink the juices at different times of the day (for example the first in the morning as soon as you wake up or in the middle of the morning, the second in the middle of the afternoon) and choose the normal or vegan dishes: Sirt omelettes, Sirt and baked chicken breast, walnut and parsley pesto and red onion salad or Walldorf salad (vegan dish) and baked eggplant wedges together with walnut and parsley pesto and tomato salad (vegan dish).

During the second phase, there are no calorie restrictions but indications on which Sirt foods must be eaten to consolidate weight loss and not run the risk of getting the lost kilograms back.

Second Phase: Maintenance

Congratulations! You have finished the first "hardcore" week. The second phase is easier and is the actual incorporation of sirtuin-filled food selections to your everyday Diet or meals. You can call this the "maintenance stage."

By doing so, your body will undergo the fat-burning stage and muscle gain plus a boost on your immune system and overall health.

For this phase, you can now have 3 balanced Sirt food-filled meals each day plus 1 green juice a day.

There is no "dieting," but more on choosing healthier alternatives with adding Sirt food in each meal as much as possible.

I will be providing some recipes for tasty dishes with Sirt food inclusion to give you further an idea of how exciting and healthy this diet journey is.

Now you move back up to a regular calorie intake with the aim to keep your weight loss steady and your Sirt food intake high. You should have experienced some degree of weight loss by now, but you should also feel trimmer and re-invigorated.

Phase 2 lasts for 14 days. During this time, you eat 3 sirt food rich meals, 1 sirt food green juice, and up to 2 optional Sirt food bite snacks. Strict calorie-counting is actively discouraged – if you follow the recommendations and eat balanced meals of reasonable portions, you shouldn't feel hungry or be consuming too much.

You should consume the same beverages you were drinking in phase 1, with the slight chance that you are welcome to enjoy the occasional glass of red wine (don't drink more than 3 per week).

Chapter 7: How to Build Your Perfect Diet

The Perfect Body Diet

- Calculate and know the right goal weight for your body.

- Determine which diet is best for you.

- Maintain and commit yourself.

What's Your Perfect Weight?

Your ideal body might be inspired by a picture you saw on a magazine cover—or by your too-skinny friend who eats bowl after bowl of New York Super Fudge Chunk and never gains an ounce. But here's what you need to remember: Your body is unique, and you need to find a realistic number that is accessible for you. Your body weight will take into account your height, bone structure, muscle mass, age, and breast size, as well as your genes. Before we do anything else, we need to figure out exactly what number you should be aiming for.

Another way to judge fullness is to keep in mind how many calories and what quantities of protein, carbs, and fats are in your food. If you know the value of the food you're putting into your body, you will be able to gauge whether it will fill you up for the long haul or for only an hour or two. For example, Tristan used to eat ½ cup of raspberries and a stick of string cheese for her mid-afternoon snack at 3:00 p.m. She thought she was doing her body a favor because the snack only contained about 100 calories, 7 grams of protein, 7 grams of carbs, and 4 grams of fat. However, she felt incredibly hungry and empty by 5:00 p.m. In truth, her snack was not substantial enough to keep her full for more than 2 hours. A full cup of berries, a stick of regular-fat string cheese, and 1½ ounces of nuts would better satisfy her because it has more calories, protein, carbs, and fat.

No matter what the underlying cause of your hunger, the solution to achieving your perfect body is to keep hunger from controlling you. You need to learn how to disregard the psychological and physiological cues and take back control over what you eat. That way, the nutrients you take in will be absorbed into your bloodstream at a steady rate, and you will no longer be a slave to hunger. Just switching to eating five or six small meals throughout the day will have a big impact. It will help you decide when to eat without relying on hunger as a cue, and at the same time, you'll always feel full.

What to Eat: Perfect Carbs, Fats, and Proteins

When you eat foods that contain starch or sugar, your stomach and intestines break them down into individual sugar units. These single sugar molecules are easily absorbed through the intestinal wall into the bloodstream, where they can provide energy (in the form of blood glucose/sugar) if you need it. If you don't need the energy right away, or if you don't need all of it at that moment, then the sugars are stored in your muscles in a form called glycogen. However, since you have only a limited amount of muscle space in which to store glycogen, the liver will convert most excess sugar into body fat. That's what you're trying to get rid of.

Carbohydrate foods that contain more fiber than sugar and starch aren't broken down as easily and have less chance to affect your body fat levels. So, the type of carbohydrate foods you eat is important because it influences how much body fat you have.

Sugars and starches are quick digesting and referred to as simple carbohydrates. Foods that contain simple carbs are mostly the human-made variety: high-sugar breakfast cereals, granola bars, and candy. Fruit juices also contain a lot of simple carbohydrates. Because simple carbs provide glucose in quantities too large to be used right away for energy, they are more likely to be stored as body fat.

Foods that are broken down slowly, thanks to a high amount of fiber, are called complex carbohydrates. These foods are less likely to be stored as body fat because they deliver a smaller, steadier influx of energy that your body will use as its provided.

Meal Setting

The Sirt food Diet is separated into two fundamental stages or phases.

Stage one goes on for seven days. For the initial three days, the diet calls for expending three sirt food green juices and one feast rich in sirt foods—for a sum of 1,000 calories for every day. Days four through seven, each comprise two green juices and two dinners—for an aggregate of 1,500 calories every day. This is the piece of the arrangement wherein Goggins and Matten guarantee you can "shed seven pounds in seven days."

Stage Two is a 14-day support stage intended to "assist you with getting more fit consistently." You can have three sirt food-rich dinners in addition to one green juice every day.

The Perfect Body Exercise Program

Let's tackle the "why" first. Lots of diets work well in the short term. You reduce the number of calories you eat and pretty quickly start to notice that your tummy is a little tighter, and your hips aren't quite as broad. But often, something strange soon starts to happen: Even though you're sticking to your new lower-calorie diet, your weight loss slows to a crawl—and then stops completely. Instead of being motivated to continue, you feel hungry, cranky, and frustrated (which, trust us, is not the formula for successful weight loss).

It turns out there's a reason this happens. Your body is pretty smart: When you eat fewer calories than it needs to maintain its weight, your body thinks it's starving and responds by lowering its metabolic rate, reducing the number of calories you burn. So now you have to eat even less just to avoid putting the pounds back on—and forget about losing more weight.

We know what you're thinking: Damned if you diet, damned if you don't.

This is why exercise is so important for weight loss and, more important, for fat loss. Regular exercise keeps your metabolism running at a high level, which allows those pounds and fat stores to keep dropping off. But exercise and what you might consider being physical activity are really two different things. Physical activity is any movement that expends energy. It's usually related to everyday tasks, such as cleaning the house or mowing the lawn. While you work up a sweat doing these, we don't consider them to be exercise, which is a structured physical activity that is performed with intensity for a specified duration of time. Examples of exercise include a basketball game, mountain biking, or a weight-lifting workout. Exercise is performed specifically to increase physical fitness, which is what we're here to do.

Maintain and Commit Yourself

From here on out, your job is simply to hold on to that perfect body. Now don't get us wrong: That doesn't mean you can slide back into your old eating and (non)exercise habits. Too many women do that, which is why 95 percent of the people who lose weight end up slowly gaining it back once they go off their diets. But this is where the Women's Health Perfect Body Diet is different. Because you tailored a plan to your individual shape and body tendencies, you'll be able to follow it long after the initial eight weeks are up. You'll still see benefits and weight loss without the usual weight regain. You haven't just changed your body; you've changed your lifestyle —and your new lifestyle is going to keep your old body a thing of the past.

There are a few things to focus on as you go forward. For starters, stick with your eating plan. You've determined what types of foods are best for your body, and you have the proof right in front of you: You look better, you feel better, and your health has improved. Don't stop eating according to the plan just because you've reached your weight-loss goal.

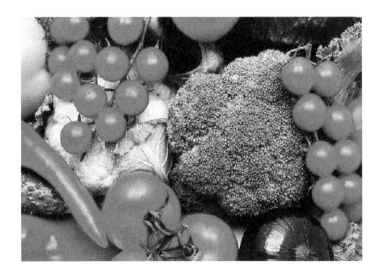

Chapter 8: Maintenance

Managing your weight with the Sirt lifestyle after the first two phases is quite simple. It would be best if you generally consumed around whatever a number of calories are recommended for your specific gender, weight, height, and activity level. You can learn this calorie recommendation from your doctor or online calorie/BMI calculators. Thankfully, you don't have to try to force yourself to stay within a certain number of calories. While you don't want to overdo this frequently by consuming too many high-calorie foods, as this can result in weight gain, it is natural for some days to be over your calorie count and other days under it. During this phase, you don't have to push yourself to stay within a set range; you can easily take things. Maybe you will occasionally allow yourself special treats of your favorite high-calorie or junk foods if it is a special occasion such as a date night or holiday.

During this phase, you should continue to drink one green juice a day, to ensure you are getting enough sirtuins. By this point, it should also be easy to include sirtuin-rich foods in all your meals, as you have learned how to do so through phases one and two.

Achieving your objectives can only prove that this diet works. So, the first phase worked like a charm for you. Even though you don't want to lose any more weight, you can stick to the maintenance phase for a long time.

You will find that exercising will become more comfortable as you lose weight and gain energy, and it will help you maintain weight.

While during the first phase of the diet, you should stick with moderate exercises and focus on not pushing your limits. Your body will adjust to the restriction in calories; later on, you can up the difficulty. Of course, you still want to pay attention to your body's needs and follow its signals for when you should rest, but if you're going to increase your abilities through exercise, you will have to push your limits to a certain extent. To do this without illness or injury, you should always discuss the matter with your doctor.

While you may choose to train and exercise alone, consider taking some classes at a local gym. By accepting these classes or hiring a personal trainer, you can have a workout fit for your individual needs and abilities, and a person guiding you that is skilled in avoiding injury.

Remember to always consume protein after your workout, ideally about an hour afterward. This is important, as the protein will strengthen and repair your muscles, reduce soreness, and boost recovery. There are many ways you can consume this protein, whether with a low-sugar soy protein shake or by merely timing your breakfast or lunch appropriately.

With the Sirt diet, you can lose weight, change your eating habits for the better, become more active, and overall improve your lifestyle. Starting the Sirt diet can be a challenge at first, as all significant life changes are, but it is well worth the effort. Listen to your body, be kind to yourself, and enjoy the benefits.

Chapter 9: Easy to Make Recipes – Breakfast Recipes

Soy Berry Smoothie

Preparation Time: 5 minutes

Cooking Time: 0 minute

Serving: 1

Ingredients:

1 cup fresh strawberries/blueberries (or frozen)

1 cup unsweetened vanilla soymilk

Directions:

Blend or blitz all the ingredients. Enjoy.

Nutrition: Calories 260, 44g net carbs, 34g sugar, and 4.5g fat.

Paleolicious Smoothie Bowl

Preparation Time: 5 minutes

Cooking Time: 0 minutes

Serving: 1

Ingredients:

1-piece Banana (frozen)

1 hand Spinach

1/2 pieces Mango

1/2 pieces Avocado

7 tbsp Almond milk

For garnish:

Mango1/2 pieces

Raspberries1 hand

Grated coconut1 tbsp

Walnuts (roughly chopped)1 tbsp

Directions:

Put ingredients in a blender and mix to an even mass.

Put the mixture in a bowl and garnish with the remaining ingredients.

Of course, you can vary the garnish as you wish.

Nutrition: Calories 180, 42g net carbs, 30g sugar, and 31.5g fat.

Banana-Peanut Butter 'n Greens Smoothie

Preparation time: 5 minutes

Cooking Time: 0 minutes

Servings: 1

Ingredients:

1 cup chopped and packed Romaine lettuce

1 frozen medium banana

1 tbsp all-natural peanut butter

1 cup cold almond milk

Directions:

In a heavy-duty blender, add all ingredients.

Puree until smooth and creamy.

Serve and enjoy.

Nutrition: Calories: 349.3, Fat:9.7 g, Carbs:57.4 g, Protein:8.1 g, Sugars:4.3 g, Sodium:151 mg

Fruity Tofu Smoothie

Preparation time: 5 minutes

Cooking Time: 0 minutes

Servings: 2

Ingredients:

1 cup ice cold water

1 cup packed spinach

¼ cup frozen mango chunks

½ cup frozen pineapple chunks

1 tbsp chia seeds

1 container silken tofu

1 frozen medium banana

Directions:

Add all ingredients in a blender until smooth and creamy.

Evenly divide into two glasses, serve and enjoy.

Nutrition: Calories: 175, Fat:3.7 g, Carbs:33.3 g, Protein:6.0 g, Sugars:16.3 g, Sodium:24.1 mg

Green Vegetable Smoothie

Preparation time: 5 minutes

Cooking Time: 0 minutes

Servings: 4

Ingredients:

1 cup cold water

½ cup strawberries

2 oz. baby spinach

1 lemon juice

1 tbsp fresh mint

1 banana

½ cup blueberries

Directions:

Put the ingredients in a blender.

Nutrition: Calories: 52, Fat:2 g, Carbs:12 g, Protein:1 g, Sugars:18 g, Sodium:36 mg

Creamy Oats, Greens & Blueberry Smoothie

Preparation time: 4 minutes

Cooking Time: 0 minutes

Servings: 1

Ingredients:

1 cup cold fat-free milk

1 cup salad greens

½ cup fresh frozen blueberries

½ cup frozen cooked oatmeal

1 tbsp sunflower seeds

Directions:

In a blender, put all ingredients until smooth and creamy.

Serve and enjoy.

Nutrition: Calories: 280, Fat: 6.8 g, Carbs: 44.0 g, Protein: 14.0 g, Sugars: 32 g, Sodium: 242 mg

Chapter 10: East to Make Recipes – Lunch Bites

Potato Bites

Preparation time: 10 minutes

Cooking time: 20 minutes

Servings: 3

Ingredients:

1 potato, sliced

2 bacon slices, already cooked and crumbled

1 small avocado, pitted and cubed

Cooking spray

Directions:

Spread potato slices on a lined baking sheet, spray with cooking oil, introduce in the oven at 350° F, bake for 20 minutes, arrange on a platter, top each slice with avocado and crumbled bacon and serve as a snack.

Nutrition: Calories 180, fat 4, fiber 1, carbs 8, protein 6g

Salmon and Quinoa Salad

Preparation time: 10 minutes

Cooking time: 20 minutes

Servings: 4

Ingredients:

1 cup white quinoa, rinsed

1 bunch kale, torn

2 tbsp lemon juice

1 carrot, sliced

2 cups water

2 garlic cloves, minced

1 tbsp olive oil

A pinch of salt and black pepper

2 cups canned chickpeas, drained and rinsed

¼ cup dried currants

1 tbsp hemp seeds

4 salmon fillets, skin-on and boneless

For the sauce:

½ cup water

¼ cup tahini paste

1 tbsp lemon juice

½ cup coconut cream

Directions:

Put the quinoa with 2 cups water in a pot then bring to a simmer over medium heat, cook for 15 minutes, set aside for another 10 minutes to cool and then fluff with a fork. In a salad bowl, mix the cooked quinoa with carrot, garlic, chickpeas, currants, kale, lemon juice and hemp seed and toss. In another bowl, combine ½ cup water with tahini, 1 tbsp lemon juice, and coconut cream, whisk well and pour over the quinoa mix. Toss the mix and set aside. Heat pan with olive oil (medium-high heat), add the salmon, season with salt and pepper and cook for 3-4 minutes on each side. Divide between plates, add the quinoa mix on the side, and serve.

Nutrition: Calories 211, fat 14, fiber: 10, carbs 16, protein 12g

Avocado and Salmon Salad Buffet

Preparation Time: 15 minutes

Cooking Time: 0 minutes

Servings: 4

Ingredients:

1/2 pieces Cucumber

2-piece Avocado

½ pieces Red onion

1 cup mixed salad

4 slices smoked salmon

Directions:

Cut the cucumber and avocado (cubes) and chop the onion.

Spread the lettuce leaves on deep plates and spread the cucumber, avocado, and onion over the lettuce.

Season with salt and pepper or you may also add a little olive oil.

Place smoked salmon slices on top and serve.

Nutrition: Calories: 143, Carbs: 11.6g, Fat: 3.4g, Protein: 28.3g

Cucumber Salad with Lime and Coriander

Preparation Time: 10 minutes

Cooking Time: 0 minutes

Serving: 1

Ingredients:

1-piece Red onion

2 pieces Cucumber

2 pieces Lime (juice)

2 tbsp fresh coriander

1 tps olive oil

Directions:

Cut the onion into rings and thinly slice the cucumber. Chop the coriander finely.

Place the onion rings in a bowl and season with about half a tbsp of salt.

Rub it in well and then fill the bowl with water.

Pour off the water and then rinse the onion rings thoroughly (in a sieve).

Put the cucumber slices together with onion, lime juice, coriander and olive oil in a salad bowl and stir everything well.

Season with salt.

Nutrition: Calories: 53, Carbs: 1g, Fat: 6g, Protein: 0g

Salad with salmon and caramelized chicory

Preparation time: 10 minutes

Cooking Time: 8 minutes

Serving: 1

Ingredients:

2 tsp parsley

juice of a quarter of a lemon

1 tbsp capers

extra virgin olive oil

1/4 avocado sliced

7 tbsp cherry tomatoes halved

4 tsp red onions, sliced

3 tbsp rocket salad

1 tsp celery leaves

10 tbsp salmon fillet without skin

2 tsp of brown sugar

1 chicory, halved lengthwise

Directions:

Preheat oven to 425° F.

The dressing: Mix parsley, lemon juice, capers and 2 tsp of olive oil in a blender to a sauce.

Mix avocado, tomato, red onion and celery green for the salad. Rub the salmon with a little oil and fry it briefly on both sides in a coated pan. Then place in the oven for about five minutes.

Mix 1 tsp of olive oil with the brown sugar and rub it into the chicory's cut surfaces. Fry on medium heat for 3 minutes in a pan.

Mix the salad with the dressing and serve with salmon and chicory.

Nutrition: Calories: 550, Carbs: 35g, Fat: 20g, Protein: 30g

Shrimp, Tomato and Dates Salad

Preparation time: 10 minutes

Cooking time: 0 minutes

Servings: 4

Ingredients:

1-pound shrimp, cooked, peeled and deveined

2 cups baby spinach

2 tbsp walnuts, chopped

1 cup cherry tomatoes, halved

1 tbsp lemon juice

½ cup dates, chopped

2 tbsp avocado oil

Directions:

In a salad bowl, mix the shrimp with the spinach, walnuts, and the other ingredients, toss and serve.

Nutrition: Calories: 72, Carbs: 0g, Fat: 0g, Protein: 0g

Chapter 11: Easy to Make Recipes – Main Meals

Curry Chicken with Pumpkin Spaghetti

Preparation time: 30 minutes

Cooking time: 2-4 hours

Servings: 4

Ingredients:

1.1 lbs Chicken breast

2 tsp Chili powder

1-piece Onion

1 clove Garlic

2 tsp Ghee

3 tbsp Curry powder

18-ounce Coconut milk

7-ounce Pineapple

7-ounce Mango

1-piece Red pepper

1-piece Butternut squash

4 tsp Spring onion

4 tsp fresh coriander

Directions:

Cut the chicken (strips) and season with pepper, salt and chili powder. Then put the chicken in the slow cooker.

Finely chop the onion and garlic and lightly fry with 2 tsp of ghee. Then add the curry powder.

Deglaze with the coconut milk after a minute. Add the sauce to the slow cooker along with the pineapple, mango cubes, and chopped peppers and let it cook for 2 to 4 hours.

Cut the pumpkin into long pieces and make spaghetti out of it with a spiralizer.

Briefly fry the pumpkin spaghetti in the pan and spread the chicken curry on top.

Garnish with thinly sliced spring onions and chopped coriander.

Nutrition: Calories: 357, Carbs: 20g, Fat: 21g, Protein: 25g

French Style Chicken Thighs

Preparation time: 20 minutes

Cooking time: 45 minutes

Servings: 3

Ingredients:

1.5 lbs Chicken leg

1 tbsp Olive oil

2 pieces Onion

4 pieces Carrot

2 cloves Garlic

8 stems Celery

4 tsp fresh rosemary

4 tsp Fresh thyme

4 tsp fresh parsley

Directions:

Season the chicken with olive oil, pepper and salt and rub it into the meat.

Roughly cut onions, carrots, garlic, and celery and add to the slow cooker. Sprinkle the chicken with a few sprigs of rosemary, thyme, and parsley on top. Cook for at least four hours.

Nutrition: Calories: 329, Carbs: 7g, Fat: 20g, Protein: 32g

Roast Beef with Grilled Vegetables

Preparation time: 10 minutes

Cooking time: 30 minutes

Servings: 3

Ingredients:

1.1 lbs Roast beef

1 clove Garlic (pressed)

1 tsp fresh rosemary

2 cups Broccoli

1 cup Carrot

2 cups Zucchini

4 tbsp Olive oil

Directions:

Rub the roast beef with freshly ground pepper, salt, garlic and rosemary.

Heat grill pan (high heat) and grill the roast beef for about 20 minutes.

Then wrap in aluminum foil and let it rest for a while.

Cut the roast beef into thin slices before serving.

Preheat the oven to 401° F. Put all the vegetables in a baking dish.

Drizzle the vegetables with olive oil and put curry powder and or chili flakes. Bake for 30 minutes.

Nutrition: Calories: 110, Carbs: 16g, Fat: 2g, Protein: 8g

Casserole with Spinach and Eggplant

Preparation time: 20 minutes

Cooking time: 40 minutes

Servings: 2

Ingredients:

1-piece Eggplant

2 pieces Onion

Olive oil 3 tbsp

2 cups Spinach

4 pcs Tomatoes

2 pcs Egg

½ tbsp Almond milk

2 tsp Lemon juice

4 tbsp Almond flour

Directions:

Preheat the oven to 392° F.

Cut the eggplants, onions, and tomatoes into slices and sprinkle salt on the eggplant slices.

Brush the eggplants and onions with olive oil and fry them in a grill pan.

Shrink the spinach in a large saucepan over moderate heat and drain in a sieve.

Put the vegetables in a greased baking dish: first the eggplant, then the spinach and then the onion and the tomato. Repeat this again.

Whisk eggs with almond milk, lemon juice, salt and pepper and pour over the vegetables.

Sprinkle almond flour over the dish and bake in the oven for 40 minutes.

Nutrition: Calories: 100, Carbs: 10g, Fat: 12g, Protein 9g

Vegetarian Paleo Ratatouille:

Preparation Time: 10 Minutes

Cooking Time: 50 Minutes

Serving: 4

Ingredients:

1 cup Tomato cubes

½ pieces Onion

2 cloves Garlic

¼ tsp dried oregano

¼ TL Chili flakes

2 tbsp Olive oil

1-piece Eggplant

1-piece Zucchini

1-piece hot peppers

1 tsp dried thyme

Directions:

Preheat the oven (673° F) and lightly grease a round shape.

Finely chop the onion and garlic.

Mix the tomato cubes with garlic, onion, oregano and chilli flakes, season with salt and pepper, and put on the bottom of the baking dish.

Use a mandolin, a cheese slicer or a sharp knife to cut the eggplant, zucchini and hot pepper into thin slices.

Put the vegetables in a bowl.

Drizzle the remaining olive oil on the vegetables and sprinkle with thyme, salt and pepper.

Cover the baking dish with a piece of parchment paper and bake in the oven for 45 to 55 minutes.

Nutrition: Calories: 180, Carbs: 29g, Fat: 5g, Protein: 8g

Vegan Thai Green Curry

Preparation time: 10 minutes

Cooking time: 60/70 minutes

Servings: 2

Ingredients:

2 pieces green chillies

1-piece Onion

1 clove Garlic

1 tsp fresh ginger (grated)

4 tsp fresh coriander

1 tsp Ground caraway

1-piece Lime (juice)

1 tsp Coconut oil

2 cups Coconut milk

1-piece Zucchini

1-piece Broccoli

1-piece Red pepper

For the cauliflower rice:

1 tsp Coconut oil

1-piece Cauliflower

Directions:

For cauliflower rice, cut the cauliflower into florets and place in the food processor. Pulse briefly until rice has formed. Put aside.

Cut the green peppers, onions, garlic, fresh ginger and coriander into large pieces and combine with the caraway seeds and the juice of 1 lime in a food processor or blender and mix to an even paste.

Heat a pan (medium heat) with a tsp of coconut oil and gently fry the pasta. Deglaze with coconut milk and add to the slow cooker.

Cut the zucchini into pieces, the broccoli in florets, the peppers into cubes and put in the slow cooker. Simmer for 4 hours.

Briefly heat the cauliflower rice in 1 tsp of coconut oil, season with a little salt and pepper in a pan over medium heat.

Nutrition: Calories: 232, Carbs: 40g, Fat: 10g, Protein: 10g

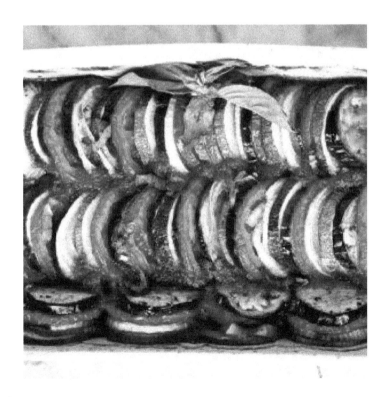

Chapter 12: Easy to Make Recipes – Dessert

Raw vegan coffee cashew cream cake

Preparation time: 10 minutes

Cooking time: 0 minutes

Servings: 4

Ingredients:

Coffee cashew cream

2 cups raw cashews

1 tsp. of ground vanilla bean

3 tbsps. melted coconut oil

¼ cup raw honey

1/3 cup very strong coffee or triple espresso shot

Directions:

Blend all ingredients for the cream, pour it onto the crust and refrigerate.

Garnish with coffee beans.

Nutrition: calories 120, fat 3g, fiber 4g, protein 3g

Raw vegan chocolate cashew truffles

Preparation time: 10 minutes

Cooking time: 0 minutes

Servings: 4

Ingredients:

1 cup ground cashews

1 tsp. of ground vanilla bean

½ cup of coconut oil

¼ cup raw honey

2 tbsp flax meal

2 tbsp hemp hearts

2 tbsp cacao powder

Directions:

Mix all ingredients and make truffles. Sprinkle coconut flakes on top.

Nutrition: Calories: 190, Carbs 20g. Dietary Fiber 2g. Sugar 5g. Fat 4g. Saturated 1g

Raw vegan double almond raw chocolate tart

Preparation time: 10 minutes

Cooking time: 35 minutes

Servings: 4

Ingredients:

1½ cups of raw almonds

¼ cup of coconut oil, melted

1 tbsp raw honey or royal jelly

8 ounces dark chocolate, chopped

1 cup of coconut milk

½ cup almond slivers

Directions:

Crust:

Ground almonds and add melted coconut oil, raw honey and combine.

Using a spatula, spread this mixture into the tart or pie pan.

Filling:

Put the chopped chocolate in a bowl, heat coconut milk and pour over chocolate and whisk together.

Pour filling into tart shell.

Refrigerate.

Toast almond slivers chips and sprinkle over tart.

Nutrition: Calories: 240, Carbs 40g. Dietary Fiber, 2.5g. Sugar 3g. Fat 3g. Saturated 1g

Raw vegan "peanut" butter truffles

Preparation time: 10 minutes

Cooking time: 30 minutes

Servings: 4

Ingredients:

5 tbsp sunflower seed butter

1 tbsp coconut oil

1 tbsp raw honey

1 tsp. ground vanilla bean

¾ cup almond flour

1 tbsp flaxseed meal

Pinch of salt

1 tbsp cacao butter

hemp hearts (optional)

¼ cup super-foods chocolate

Directions:

Mix until all ingredients are incorporated.

Roll the dough into 1-inch balls, place them on parchment paper and refrigerate for half an hour (yield about 14 truffles).

Dip each truffle in the melted superfoods chocolate, one at the time.

Place them back on the pan with parchment paper or coat them in cocoa powder or coconut flakes.

Nutrition: Calories: 578, Carbs41g. Dietary Fiber 2g. Sugar2g. Fat 4g. Saturated 1g

Frozen raw blackberry cake

Preparation time: 10 minutes

Cooking time: 45 minutes

Servings: 4

Ingredients:

Crust:

3⁄4 cup shredded coconut

15 dried dates soaked in hot water and drained

1/3 cup pumpkin seeds

1⁄4 cup of coconut oil

Middle filling

Coconut whipped cream - see Coconut Whipped Cream recipes.

Top filling:

1 pound of frozen blackberries

3-4 tbsps. raw honey

1⁄4 cup of coconut cream

2 egg whites

Directions:

Grease the cake tin with coconut oil and mix all base ingredients in the blender until you get a sticky ball.

Press the base mixture in a cake tin.

Freeze.

Make Coconut Whipped Cream.

Process berries and add honey, coconut cream and egg whites.

Pour middle filling - Coconut Whipped Cream in the tin and spread evenly.

Freeze.

Pour top filling - berries mixture-in the tin, spread, decorate with blueberries and almonds and return to freezer.

Nutrition: Calories: 62, Carbs39g. Dietary Fiber2g. Sugar2g. Fat4g. Saturated 1g

Raw Vegan Chocolate Hazelnuts Truffles

Preparation time: 10 minutes

Cooking time: 30 minutes

Servings: 4

Ingredients:

1 cup ground almonds

1 tsp. ground vanilla bean

½ cup of coconut oil

½ cup mashed pitted dates

12 whole hazelnuts

2 tbsps. cacao powder

Directions:

Mix all ingredients and make truffles with one whole hazelnut in the middle.

Nutrition: Calories: 190, Carbs40g. Dietary Fiber 3g. Sugar 2g. Fat 4g. Saturated 1g

Chapter 13: Easy to Make Recipes – Snack

Fruity Granola Bars

Preparation time: 25 minutes

Cooking Time: 30 minutes

Serving: 24

Ingredients:

¾ cup packed brown sugar

½ cup honey

¼ cup of water

1 tsp salt

½ cup of cocoa butter

3 cups rolled oats

1 cup walnuts, chopped

1 cup ground buckwheat

¼ cup sesame seeds

½ cup dried strawberries or mixed fruits

½ cup raisins

½ cup Medjool dates, chopped

Directions:

In a large pan, combine sugar, cocoa butter, honey, water, and salt. Bring to a simmer and cook for 5 minutes.

Stir in oats, walnuts, ground buckwheat, and sesame seeds. Cook, frequently stirring, for 15 minutes. Remove from heat and add dried fruits.

Pour into a large baking sheet lined with wax or parchment paper. Press firmly to create an even layer.

Score deeply into bars roughly 2" wide by 4" tall.

Allow cooling for 30 minutes before breaking or cutting along score lines. Store in an air tight container.

Nutrition: calories 130, fat 4, fiber 5, carbs 15, protein 15g

Cardamom Granola Bars

Preparation time: 10 minutes

Baking time: 30 minutes

Cooking time: 30 minutes cooling

Serving: 18

Ingredients:

2 cups rolled oats

½ cup raisins

½ cup walnuts, chopped and toasted

1 ½ tsp ground cardamom

6 tbsp cocoa butter

1/3 cup packed brown sugar

3 tbsp honey

Coconut oil, for greasing pan

Directions:

Preheat oven to 350° F.

Line a 9-inch square pan with foil, extending the foil over the sides. Grease the foil with coconut oil.

Mix the oats, raisins, walnuts and cardamom in a large bowl.

Heat the cocoa butter, brown sugar and honey in a saucepan until the butter melts and begins to bubble.

Pour this mixture over the dry ingredients and mix until well coated. Transfer to the prepared pan and press evenly with a spatula.

Bake for 30 minutes or until the top is golden brown.

Allow cooling for 30 minutes. Using the foil, lift the granola out of the pan and place on cutting board.

Nutrition: calories 140, fat 4, fiber 6, carbs 10, protein 15g

Coconut Brownie Bites

Preparation time: 15 minutes

Cooking time: 30 minutes – 2 hours

Serving: 24-30

Ingredients:

2 ½ cups walnuts

¼ cup almonds

2 ½ cups Medjool dates

¼ cup unsweetened cocoa powder

1 tsp vanilla extract

¼ tsp of sea salt

¼ cup unsweetened desiccated or shredded coconut

Directions

Place everything in a food processor and blend until well combined.

Roll into 1" balls.

Roll balls in coconut until well-covered and place on a wax paper-lined baking sheet.

Freeze for 30 minutes or refrigerate for up to 2 hours.

Nutrition: calories 120, fat 3, fiber 5, carbs 15, protein 15g

Tortilla Chips and Fresh Salsa

Preparation time: 10 minutes

Cooking time: 10 minutes

Serving: 4

Ingredients:

4 whole wheat flour tortillas

2 tbsp extra virgin olive oil

4 Roma tomatoes, diced

1 small red onion, finely diced

1 Bird's Eye chilli pepper, finely diced

2 tsp parsley, finely chopped

2 tsp cilantro, finely chopped

1 lime, juiced

Salt and pepper to taste

Directions:

Preheat oven to 350° F.

Using a pastry brush, coat one side of each tortilla in olive oil.

With a sharp knife or pizza cutter, divide each tortilla into 8 wedges. Spread tortillas over a large baking sheet in a single layer. Use more than one baking sheet if necessary.

Bake for 8 – 10 minutes, flipping halfway through until both sides are golden brown and your chips are crispy.

While the chips are baking, combine tomatoes, red onion, chili pepper, parsley, cilantro and lime juice and mix well.

Serve salsa with the chips.

Nutrition: calories 140, fat 4, fiber 5, carbs 15, protein 15g

Garlic Baked Kale Chips

Preparation time: 30 minutes

Cooking time: 25/30 minutes

Serving: 2

Ingredients:

1 bunch kale leaves

½ tbsp extra-virgin olive oil

1 tsp garlic powder

1/8 tsp cayenne powder

¼ tsp fine salt

Directions:

Preheat oven to 300° F and cover a large baking sheet with parchment paper.

Remove the stems from your kale and tear up into large pieces.

Wash and spin the leaves until thoroughly dry, using a paper towel to pat dry if necessary.

Place kale leaves in a large bowl and massage the olive oil thoroughly into each leaf.

Combine garlic, cayenne and salt in a small bowl and mix well.

Sprinkle seasoning over kale and toss to distribute.

Spread kale in a single layer over the baking sheet.

Bake for 10 minutes, rotate the pan and bake for another 12-15 minutes more until the kale just begins to get crispy. The leaves will shrink and need to cool at least 5 minutes after being taken out of the oven to crisp properly.

Nutrition: calories 150, fat 6, fiber 5, carbs 20, protein 20g

Cauliflower Nachos

Preparation time: 5 minutes

Cooking time: 20 - 25 minutes

Serving: 4

Ingredients:

2 tbsp extra virgin olive oil

½ tsp onion powder

½ tsp turmeric

½ tsp ground cumin

1 large head cauliflower

¾ cup shredded cheddar cheese

½ cup tomato, diced

¼ cup red bell pepper, diced

¼ cup red onion, diced

½ Bird's Eye chilli pepper, finely diced

¼ cup parsley, finely diced

Pinch of salt

Directions:

Preheat oven to 400° F.

Mix onion powder, cumin, turmeric and olive oil.

Core cauliflower and slice into ½" thick rounds.

Coat the cauliflower with the olive oil mixture and bake for 15 – 20 minutes.

Top with shredded cheese & bake for an additional 3 – 5 minutes, until cheese is melted.

In a bowl, combine tomatoes, bell pepper, onion, chili and parsley with a pinch of salt.

Top cooked cauliflower with salsa and serve.

Nutrition: calories 150, fat 4, fiber 3, carbs 15, protein 17g

Chapter 14: Celebrities Who Are Funs of the Sirtfood Diet

The sirt food diet has been endorsed by James Haskell, Jodie Kidd, and Lorraine Pascale. This has increased its popularity.

A TV chef calls the Sirt food Diet a "non-faddy diet" that offers health benefits and weight loss results. Best of all, it doesn't feel like dieting because you're eating delicious food.

The Sirt food Diet may become a weight-loss choice for the ones who already think of New Year's resolutions because celebrities like Adele and Pippa Middleton have used it. They assumed a slim body as a result of following this trend.

As mentioned earlier, the U.K. nutrition specialists, Aidan Goggins, and Glen Matten had developed the Sirt food Diet; the weight loss plan is designed to support the "skinny gene." It has the SIRT1 gene name, and Sirt food Diet even claims to help with inflammation and weight gain.

Adele, a British celebrity, is one popular case who has lost her weight through the Sirt food diet. It was interesting Adele has lost weight through a diet that requires red wine and chocolate.

The 31-year-old singer debuted his slimmer figure this fall to fans all over the country. Over her holidays, she continued to drop pounds and even worried some viewers that she was too slim in recent pictures of paparazzi.

By hiring a personal trainer and adopting a Sirt food diet, the brit would also have lost almost 50 pounds to a meal plan that it had been related to after losing weight in 2016.

And Adele is not the one who focuses on foods that control one's metabolism with the buzzy diet. Pippa Middleton younger sister of the Duchess of Cambridge is said to be a fan, and the program for food was Google's seventh most searched diet in 2019.

Aidan Goggins & Glen Matten, the U.K nutritionists, and founders of sirt food released a guide and a recipe book in 2016. The diet was based on sirt foods. The diet concentrates on sirtuins or proteins in your body, which, among other things, specialize in cellular health and metabolism. Foods such as kale, extra-virgin olive oil, and buckwheat, matcha, bleeding, and arugula, sirtuins may be contained. Red wine, coffee, and dark chocolate are the sweet surprises of the menu. Food is no beast. Meat is not a monster.

The most famous argument is that it can motivate you to lose up to seven pounds a week, one of its founders, Matten told. It is also shown by Adele's transformation over the years. But this isn't a cake: For three days just 1000 calories a day are eaten by eaters— one meal filled with sirtuins and two green juices. In the next four days, an additional meal will allow up to 1.500 calories to be bumped. After that week, you can eat as much sirt food as you want. Daily exercise on a diet is also advisable.

The foods should increase muscle growth because their "skin gene" activates the effects of diet and exercise. The foods are supposed to increase muscle growth.

A nutritionist, Martha McKittrick from Manhattan, said recently that the diet she believes is "skuzzy." "Not everyone will be able to see the results from Adele," said Grace Feldberg, a registered dietitian.

However, this diet has been classified as the most searched 2019 diet for Google No. 7. According to Trudy Thelander, a co-creator of the Mediterranean diet — the original inspiration for the S diet is actually scientifically sound.

German scientific study of the benefits of a Mediterranean diet that combines two of the world's healthiest diets— the Mediterranean and Asian,' she said. "The term 'Sirt food' has come to be coined by German scientists from Kiel University."

Traditional Mediterranean and Asian diets are rich in compounds known as polyphenols of natural vegetables. The consumption by a special family of body genes called Sirtuins, which play an essential role in slowing down cell age, reducing inflammation and regulating blood sugars, of these polyphenolic foods — including extra virgin olive oil, peat, capers, green tea, and red wines. The ability of the body to burn fat can be increased.

The researchers have found that the advantages of a Mediterranean diet that activates sirtuin are similar to severe calorie limiting (such as fasting) but without having to limit calories. The results have been obtained. Their pioneering research was published in 2013." We propose that a so-called" Mediterranean "diet combining sirtuin activated food (= Sirt food) from both the Asian and Mediterranean Diets may be a very promise-oriented dietary strategy for preventing chronic conditions, ensuring that people have healthy eating and good aging." "Unlike modern, highly-processed Western diets, Mediterranean foods rely on minimum-processed foods, such as vegetables, fruit, grains, boars, nuts, olive oil, and fish. These foods are overflowing with health-promoting compounds, including omega-three fatty acids, plant chemicals, antioxidants, and dietary fiber, which are good for good health and are also great for good health. "Eating this way is not at all restrictive, but it's very enjoyable," says Dietitian Caroline Fernandes. "Some of our best food is from Mediterranean and Asian regions such as Italy, Greece, and Japan. Patients are now recommending a Mediterranean diet, and the results were highly positive. "We observed, in practice, that patients don't feel in the limited sense of the word, in a diet but are transiting to a new way of life that implies the harmonious blend of flavors, food, and seasonings."

Chapter 15: Building a Diet That Works

With the Sirt food Diet, we've done something very special.

We've taken the foremost potent Sirt foods on the earth and have woven them into a brand-new way of eating, the likes of which haven't been seen before. We've selected the "best of the best" from the healthiest diets ever known and from them created a world-beating diet.

The good news is, you don't need to suddenly adopt the healthy diet of an Okinawan or be ready to cook like an Italian mamma. That's not only wholly unrealistic but unnecessary on the Sirt food Diet. Indeed, one thing which will strike you from the list of Sirt foods is their familiarity. While you'll not currently be eating all the foods on the list, you are probably consuming some. So why are you not already losing weight?

The answer is found once we examine the various elements that the first cutting-edge nutritional science shows are needed for building a diet that works. It's about eating Sirt foods within the right quantity, variety, and form. It's about complementing Sirt food dishes with generous servings of protein than eating your meals at the most straightforward time. It's about the liberty to eat the authentic tasty foods that you enjoy within the amounts you wish.

Hitting Your Quota

Right now, most of the people don't consume nearly enough Sirt foods to elicit a potent fat-burning and health-boosting effect.

When researchers checked out the consumption of 5 essential sirtuin-activating nutrients (quercetin, myricetin, kaempferol, luteolin, and apigenin) within the US diet, they found individual daily intakes to be a miserly 13 milligrams per day. In contrast, the typical Japanese intake was five times higher. Compare that with our Sirt food Diet trial, where individuals were consuming many milligrams of sirtuin-activating nutrients a day.

What we are talking about maybe a total diet revolution where we increase our daily intake of sirtuin-activating nutrients by the maximum amount as fiftyfold. While this might sound daunting or impractical, it isn't. By taking all our top Sirt foods and putting them together during a way that's compatible together with your busy life, you can also quickly and effectively reach the extent of intake needed to reap all the advantages.

The Power of Synergy

We believe it's better to eat a good range of those wonder nutrients within the sort of natural whole foods, where they coexist alongside the natural bioactive plant chemicals that act synergistically to spice up our health. We expect it's better to figure with nature instead of against it. It's, for this reason, that point and time again supplements of isolated nutrients fail to point out the benefit, yet the same nutrient, when provided within the sort of whole food, does.

Take, for instance, the classic sirtuin-activating nutrient resveratrol. In its supplement form, it's poorly absorbed; but in the natural matrix of wine, wine's bioavailability (how much the body can use) is a minimum of six-fold higher. Increase this the very fact that wine contains not only one but an entire range of sirtuin-activating polyphenols that act together to bring health benefits, including piceatannol, quercetin, myricetin, and epicatechin. Or we'd switch our attention to curcumin from turmeric.

But what makes a dietary approach special is once we begin to mix multiple Sirt foods. For instance, by adding in quercetin-rich Sirt foods, we enhance the bioavailability of resveratrol-containing foods even further. Not only this, but their actions complement one another. Both are fat busters, but there are nuances in how each of them achieves this. Resveratrol is exceptionally effective at helping to destroy existing fat cells, whereas quercetin excels in preventing new adipose cell formation. In combination, they aim fat from each side, leading to a more significant impact on fat loss than if we just ate copious amounts of one food.

The Power of Protein

It's plants that put the Sirt into the Sirt food Diet, but to reap maximum benefit, Sirt food meals should be rich in protein. A building block of a dietary protein called leucine has been shown to possess additional benefits in stimulating SIRT1 to extend fat burning and improve blood glucose control.

Eat Early

When it involves eating, our philosophy is that the earlier the higher, ideally finishing eating for the day by 7 p.m. this is often for 2 reasons. First, to reap the natural satiating effect of Sirt foods.

There are many more benefits to eating a meal, which will keep you feeling full, satisfied, and energized as you set about your day rather than spending the entire day feeling hungry only to eat and stay full as you sleep through the night.

But there's a second compelling reason: to stay eating habits in tune with your internal body clock. We all have a built-in body clock, called our biological time, which regulates many of our natural body functions consistent with the time of day.

Among other things, it influences how the body handles the food we eat. Our clocks add synchrony, primarily following the cues of the light-dark cycle of the sun. As a diurnal species, we're designed to move within the daytime instead of in the dark.

Consequently, our body clock gears us up to handle food most efficiently during the day, when it's light and that we are expected to move, and fewer so when it's dark, where we are instead primed for rest and sleep.

The problem is that many folks have "work clocks" and "social clocks" that aren't in sync with the powering down of the sun. After dark is usually the sole chance, a number of us get to eat. To a degree, we will train our body clock to sync to different schedules, like "evening chronotypes," preferring or need to move, eat, and sleep later within the day. However, living misaligned from the external light-dark cycle comes at a price.

Chapter 16: Sirt Foods

We've discovered so far that sirtuins are an ancient gene family with the power to help us burn fat, build muscle, and keep us super healthy. It is well known that by caloric restriction, fasting, and exercise, sirtuins can be turned on, but there is another innovative way to achieve this: food. We Refer to The Most Potent Foods to Cause Sirtuins As Sirtfoods.

Beyond Antioxidants

Really knowing Sirtfood's bene st requires us to think quite differently regarding foods such as fruits and vegetables, and why they are good for us. With stacks of research testifying that diets rich in fruits, vegetables, and plant foods generally slash the risk of many chronic diseases, including the biggest killers, heart disease, and cancer, there is absolutely no doubt they do. This has been put down to their rich nutrient content, such as vitamins, minerals, and, of course, antioxidants, which is probably the greatest health buzzword of the last decade. But this is a very different story we are here to tell.

The explanation Sirtfoods is so good for you has nothing to do with the nutrients that we all know so well and hear about so much. Sure, they 're all valuable things you need to get out of your diet, but with Sirtfoods there's something entirely different, and very special. In reality, what if we threw that whole way of thinking on its head and said that the reason Sirtfoods is good for you is not that they nourish the body with essential nutrients, or provide antioxidants to mop up the damaging effects of free radicals, but quite the opposite: because they are full of weak toxins? This might sound crazy in a world where almost every alleged "superfood" is aggressively marketed based on its antioxidant content. But it's a revolutionary idea, and one worth taking on.

What Doesn't Kill You Makes You Stronger?

Let's get back for a moment to the established ways to trigger sirtuins: fasting and exercise. Research has shown repeatedly, as we have seen, that the restriction of dietary energy has significant benefits for weight loss, wellbeing, and very likely longevity. Then there's exercise, with its endless benefits for both body and mind, proven out by the finding that regular exercise slashes mortality rates drastically. But what is it they have in common?

The solution lies in: heat. Both fasting and exercise are causing mild stress on the body, which encourages it to adapt by being more durable, more productive, and tighter. It is the reaction of the body to these slightly stressful stimuli — its adaptation — that in the long run, make us better, healthier, and leaner. And as we now know, sirtuins orchestrate these extremely benevolent social adaptations, which are turned on in the face of these stressors, and spark a host of beneficial changes in the body.

The scientific term used to respond to such stresses is hormesis. It's the idea that exposure to a low dose of a drug or stress that is either harmful or lethal if delivered at higher doses gives you a beneficial effect.

Enter Polyphenols

Now it is here that things really get interesting. All living organisms undergo hormesis, but what has been significantly underestimated until now is that it also involves plants. While we may not usually think of plants as being the same as other living organisms, let alone humans, we do share similar responses in terms of how we respond to our environment on a chemical level.

As mind-blowing as that sounds, it makes complete sense to think evolutionarily about it, as all living organisms have evolved to encounter and cope with common environmental stresses such as starvation, heat, lack of nutrients, and pathogens assault.

If that's difficult wrapping around your ear, get ready for the very amazing part. Reactions to plant stress are, in fact, more complex than ours. Think about it: if we're hungry and thirsty, we can go in search of food and drink; too dry, we can go out in the shade; we can see under attack. In total comparison, plants are stationary, and as such, all the severity of these physiological stresses and threats must endure. As a result, they have built a highly sophisticated stress-response mechanism over the past billion years that humble everything we can boast about. The way they do this is to produce a vast collection of natural plant chemicals — called polyphenols — that will allow them to adapt to their environment and survive successfully. We also absorb certain polyphenol nutrients when we eat these plants. Their effect is profound: they activate our own innate mechanisms to react to stress. Here we are thinking about exactly the same directions that turn on to fasting and exercise: the sirtuins.

Piggybacking on the stress-response mechanism of a plant in this way is known as xenohormesis for our own bene t. And the consequences of that are game-changing. Let the plants do the hard work, so we need not. Indeed, because of their ability to turn on the same positive changes in our cells, such as fat burning, that would be seen during fasting, these natural plant compounds are now referred to as caloric limiting mimetics. And by supplying us with more sophisticated signaling compounds than we are generating ourselves, they cause results that are superior to anything that can be obtained by fasting or exercising alone.

While all plants have these stress-response systems, only some have developed to produce remarkable amounts of polyphenols that activate the sirtuin. We are naming certain plants, Sirtfoods. Their discovery means there's now a revolutionary new way to activate your sirtuin genes instead of austere fasting regimens or arduous exercise programs: eating an abundant diet in Sirtfoods. Best of all, this one includes placing (Sirt)food on your plate, not removing it!

It's so beautifully simple and so easy it looks like a catch is needed. But it is not. This is how nature meant us to eat, rather than the rumbling stomach or calorie count of the modern diet. Many of you who have undergone such hellish diets, where the initial weight loss sites until the body rebels and the weight piles up again, would undoubtedly cringe at the thought of another false hope, another book boasting the dreaded word "d." But note this: the current dietary method is only 150 years old; Sirtfoods have been established by evolution over a billion years ago.

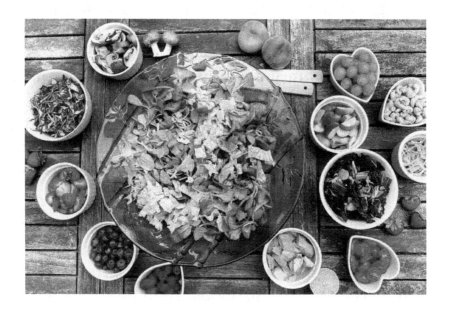

Chapter 17: Success Stories of Sirt Diet

Lorraine Pascale and the Sirtfood diet:

Lorraine Pascale is probably the world's most well-known and well-praised chef and food enthusiast. She belongs to the United Kingdom, the same country in which the Sirt food diet was first introduced. She is known as a successful supermodel when Lorraine was sixteen years old. She took care of her chronically ill mother for many years, and it was the time when she found the importance of some particular foods in the nourishment of chronically ill patients. This turned her interests in entirely different directions. She started taking an interest in cooking, and in no time, she was recognized as the most well-known and widely praised chef of the world. She has written many books on diet and foods. Over one million copies of her books were sold solely in UK, and this a huge success indeed. She is a tv host, and her shows are aired in more than 70 countries globally. The ratings of her shows are insane, and she is the most-watched chef globally.

The praise of the Sirt food diet from the guru herself was a significant breakthrough in the popularity of this dieting regime. She mentioned that the Sirt food diet is the best-known diet for her with thousands of benefits. She considers herself as the biggest fan of the Sirt food diet, which is enough with respect to the Sirt food diet.

She mentioned that the Sirt food diet was a breakthrough in achieving the best shape of her life; even this person is a supermodel herself. So notably, these statements from Lorraine Pascale are enough to establish the health benefits of the Sirt food diet.

David Haye and the Sirtfood diet:

He is one of the most dynamic boxers in history. He belongs to the UK, and he has won many titles of boxing championships. He has fought for two different weight classes in the same year and won both titles as the world's champion, thanks to the Sirt food diet and his fantastic training. David Haye is a vegan who loves vegan foods. He also holds a company that makes vegan protein powders. The number one problem of different fat loss diets is the issue related to vegan followers. Most of the ordinary fat loss diets involve a high protein diet coming from the animal source, which is, of course, big trouble for vegan lovers. Some fat loss diets are also designed for vegans, and these diets don't have any space for the meat lovers. So, this cross completion between vegan and non-vegan interest causes many issues for both categories. The Sirt food diet is unique in this regard. It contains a great variety of vegan foods as well as a perfect space for meat lovers. The diet can be modified according to personal interest, and it is a win-win situation for both. The consumer just has to stick with the basic principles of the Sirt food diet, which are very simple to follow.

This perfect diet for vegans provided significant benefits to vegan boxer David Haye during his competitions. He mentioned that the Sirt food diet provided him the most significant benefits of his career by refueling his body with a lot of energy and an easy ladder to climb up on higher weight class and winning the title against a competitor who contained 9-inch height and 45 kg weight benefit on David Haye. But his amazing skills and high energy provided by the Sirt food diet provided him with the new world heavyweight title. It is enough to describe the benefits of the Sirt food diet.

Jodie Kidd and the Sirt food diet:

Jodie Kidd is a British celebrity and supermodel who started her modeling career in just 16 years of age. At that time, she was 6 feet and 1 inch tall, with just 48 kg of body weight. Her slender physique was very famous among girls, and it was also reported that some girls turned anorexic after following her beauty standards. She took eight months from her modeling career and started eating a more caloric diet, so; size 14 was achieved in dresses worn by Jodie Kidd in those eight months. She was slender, and her most significant issue was putting on some weight rather than losing it. So, it was much different than introduced by nearly all fat loss diets. She has to put some weight while keeping the total body fat percentage low and increasing the lean muscle mass. It is not less than a fat loss challenge, and physique like Jodie Kidd had, it was even more challenging to achieve that goal. She has made multiple transformations over the course of years. She is not only a supermodel but also a fast car racer and a television host. When asked from Jodie about her perfect shape and glowing skin, she said that all credits belong to the Sirt food diet. Interestingly, the Sirt food diet was thought of as a principle fat loss diet, but Jodie used this diet to put lean muscle mass on her making her more curvaceous and healthy-looking.

Jodie said that the Sirt food diet was a game-changer for her. She followed that regime and got the best shape of her life. It was hard to put weight on her lean body, but the Sirt food diet helped her to achieve her fitness goals. She mentioned that the Sirt food diet is the key behind her good looks. These statements in favor of the Sirt food diet made this diet even more popular among the fans of Jodie, and thousands of people started using this dieting regime.

James Haskell and the Sirt food diet:

James Haskell is a former professional rugby player who played for many years as a leading rugby star from the national rugby team of the UK. He was a fantastic rugby player in both under 16 and under 18 categories. James also played as a national rugby player from Wales and Ireland. He has one of the most successful careers in rugby. James Haskell is known for his incredible athletic energy and buffed physique. He has excellent lean muscle mass on his well-ripped body and a very low-fat percentage. James has maintained his physique for years keeping the right track on his diet and eating habits. His career of rugby is charming, and now he has a high motivation to compete as a pro-MMA fighter. He will compete in the heavyweight class in May 2020 and has firm hopes about a charming career in MMA as well. James Haskell has used the Sirt food diet to keep up his body according to the standards of the heavyweight class. His statement about the Sirt food diet is very famous as he claimed that the most excellent performances of his career in the 2015 rugby world cup were due to the Sirt food diet. He trained hard and smart by keeping the Sirt food diet on the table, and this leads to incredible energy levels in his body. This statement made the Sirt food diet extremely famous among his fans as well as among his competitors, and thousands of people have followed this diet plan to achieve the best in their lives.

Sir Ben Ainslie and the Sirt food diet:

Sir Ben Ainslie is the best sailor among the history of Great Britain. He is a British national who competed in many Olympic Games and won many titles to his names. He was a sailor when he was eight years old, and he competed internationally in japan at the age of twelve. In 1996 he won the first Olympic gold medal in sailing. Ben holds medals in five different categories of sailing sports. He is one of three athletes worldwide historically who achieved this rank. Moreover, Ben is the second-best Olympic sailor who holds four gold medals in sailing sports. He is a well-known athlete of British history and praised by millions of fans. The statements of Sir Ben Ainslie about the Sirt food diet are very supportive, and Ben mentioned the Sirt food diet as the vital force behind his successful career. He said that the Sirt food diet helped him achieving the best shape of his life and the best performances of his career because of the fantastic energy and focused mind. His performances in the British-American cup are the most golden memories of his career, and he claims that the Sirt food diet helped him achieve his goals in perfection.

Adele and the Sirt food diet:

Last but not least, Adele and the Sirt food diet is probably the most fantastic story of 2020 in context to physical transformations. Adele belongs to the UK, and she has won the best singer awards throughout her career. She is no doubt one of the loveliest voices in English pop history. She has amazing vocals and a very charming personality. Adele is one of those celebrities who have struggled a lot to achieve a lean physique, but it was never easy for her before the Sirt food diet. She was chubby and got plenty of extra pounds on her body. She was quite happy with her outlook, but she is also aware of the health risks associated with high body fat percentages. Adele has reportedly lost nearly 40 pounds of extra fat from her body within a few months of following the Sirt food diet. This diet plan was also popular among many other celebrities, but the transformation shown by Adele created an incredible hype of the Sirt food diet. She now has the best shape of her life and a fantastic body, which is much leaner and healthier than before. Adele is very vocal about the health benefits of the Sirt food diet, and because of her vast transformation, the Sirt food diet is known as "The Adele Diet.

So, these statements are enough to show the benefits associated with the Sirt food diet, and when used properly, the Sirt food diet can be a great precursor behind the success of your life-changing achievements.

Chapter 18: Your 3 Weeks Meal Plan

The Sirtfood diet is based on a two-stage, three-week plan. Week one is designed to kick start the weight loss, while weeks two and three are a maintenance plan to sustain your weight loss as well as improve your overall health.

Here is a 3-week meal plan with recipes contained in this book. This plan is only to guide you in making your food choices. Feel free to go for other recipes outside the ones stated in this meal plan.

Week 1

Day 1

· Breakfast: Sirtfood green juice

· Mid-Morning: Green juice

· Lunch: Green juice

· Dinner: Roast Mackerel and simple veg Plus 20g of dark chocolate

Day 2

· Breakfast: Sirtfood green juice

· Mid-Morning: Green juice

· Lunch: Green juice

· Dinner: Tuscan bean stew Plus 20g of dark chocolate

Day 3

· Breakfast: Sirtfood green juice

· Mid-Morning: Green juice

· Lunch: Green juice

· Dinner: Chargrilled Beef with Onion Rings, Red Wine, Herb Roasted Potatoes and Garlic Kale

Plus, 20g of dark chocolate

Day 4

· Breakfast: Sirtfood green juice

· Mid-Morning: Green juice

· Lunch: Kale and Turmeric Chicken Salad and Honey Lime Dressing

· Dinner: Buckwheat Noodles with Asian King Prawn Stir-fry

Day 5

· Breakfast: Sirt Museli

· Mid-Morning: Green juice

· Lunch: Waldorf Salad

· Dinner: Sirtfood green juice

Day 6

· Breakfast: Sirtfood green juice

· Mid-Morning: Green juice

· Lunch: Miso Marinated Cod with Stir-Fried Greens and Sesame

· Dinner: Cauliflower Quinoa Meatless Meatballs in Coconut Turmeric Sauce

Day 7

· Breakfast: Smoked Salmon Omelette

· Mid-Morning: Green juice

· Lunch: Aromatic Chicken Breast with Salsa, Red Onion and Kale

· Dinner: Green juice

Phase Two – Week 2 and 3

Day 1

· Breakfast: Sirtfood Mushroom Scramble Eggs

· Mid-morning: Sirtfood green juice

· Lunch: Turmeric Zucchini Soup

· Dinner: Kale Stir-fry with Crispy Curried Tofu

· Snacks: Handful of walnuts

Day 2

· Breakfast: Turmeric Scrambled Eggs

· Mid-morning: Sirtfood green juice

· Lunch: Lentil soup

· Dinner: Chickpea Turmeric Stew with Coconut Bacon

- Snacks: 25 strawberries

Day 3

- Breakfast: Sirt Blueberry pancake
- Mid-morning: Sirtfood green juice
- Lunch: Mediterranean Hummus Pasta Salad
- Dinner: Tuscan bean stew
- Snacks: 15 blackberries

Day 4

- Breakfast: Blackcurrant and Kale Smoothie
- Mid-morning: Sirtfood green juice
- Lunch: Kale and Stilton Soup
- Dinner: Mediterranean Baked Penne
- Snacks: 10 red grapes

Day 5

- Breakfast: Green tea smoothie
- Mid-morning: Sirtfood green juice
- Lunch: Greek Salad Skewers
- Dinner: Chili Sweetcorn and Wild Garlic Fritters
- Snacks: Celery and hummus

Day 6

- Breakfast: blueberry smoothie

· Mid-morning: Sirtfood green juice

· Lunch: Veggie Chili and Baked Potato

· Dinner: Anti-Inflammatory Ginger-Turmeric Carrot Soup

· Snacks: 85% dark chocolate

Day 7

· Breakfast: Greek yogurt with chopped walnuts, 2 tsp of grated dark chocolate, and mixed berries

· Mid-morning: Sirtfood green juice

· Lunch: Chickpea and Lemony Lentil Salad with Herbs and Radish

· Dinner: Pan Fried Salmon with Caramelized Chicory, Rocket and Celery Leaf Salad

· Snacks: Mixed berries

Day 8

· Breakfast: Kale omelette

· Mid-morning: Sirtfood green juice

· Lunch: The Sirtfood's Walnut and Date Porridge

· Dinner: Edamame, Kale and Tofu Curry

Snacks: 5 dates

Day 9

· Breakfast: Sirtfood omelette

· Mid-morning: Sirtfood green juice

· Lunch: Kale Stir-fry with Crispy Curried Tofu

· Dinner: Buckwheat Kasha with Onions and Mushroom

· Snacks: 1 cup of coffee

Day 10

· Breakfast: 1 cup of green tea and scrambled eggs

· Mid-morning: Sirtfood green juice

· Lunch: Buckwheat Pancakes with Dark Chocolate Sauce, Strawberries and Crushed Walnuts

· Dinner: Strawberry Buckwheat Tabbouleh

· Snacks: 10 red grapes

Day 11

· Breakfast: Sirtfood Diet Green Juice Salad

· Mid-morning: Sirtfood green juice

· Lunch: Baked Potatoes with Spicy Chickpea Stew

· Dinner: Buckwheat Noodles with Chicken, Kale and Miso Dressing

· Snacks: 25g dark chocolate

Day 12

· Breakfast: Blueberry smoothie

· Mid-morning: Sirtfood green juice

· Lunch: Buckwheat Pasta Salad

· Dinner: Roast beef with grilled vegetables

· Snacks: 25 blueberries

Day 13

· Breakfast: Green tea smoothie

· Mid-morning: Sirtfood green juice

· Lunch: 5-Minute Air Fryer Parmesan and Feta Cheese Kale Salad

· Dinner: Sirtfood Easy Chickpea Curry and Buckwheat Noodles

· Snacks: 85% dark chocolate

Day 14

· Breakfast: Green smoothie

· Mid-morning: Sirtfood green juice

· Lunch: Buckwheat Noodles with Asian King Prawn Stir-fry

· Dinner: Ginger and Turmeric Meatballs

· Snacks: olives

Chapter 19: Sirtfood Diet Theory

The Sirtfood diet attempts to emulate the advantages of fasting diets, but without any of the drawbacks.

Many fasting diets have become popular over the past five years. The most well-known are the several variants of the intermittent fasting structure, such as the five-two diet. In the five-two menu, you fast during the weekend and usually eat during the week's working days. These diets have proven and demonstrated effects on longevity, weight loss, and overall health.

This is because these fasting diets activate the 'skinny gene' in our body. This gene causes the fat-storage processes to shut down and for the body to enter a state of 'survival' mode, which in turn causes the body to burn fat.

Burning fat is what you might expect if you necessarily start starving yourself, but another exciting effect of fasting is that your body switches from the replication of cells to the repair of cells.

Anytime cells in your body replicate, there is a small chance of your D.N.A. being damaged in the process. However, if your body repairs dying and older cells, there is no risk of D.N.A. damage, which is why fasting is associated with a lower prevalence of degenerative diseases, such as Alzheimer's.

However, the problem with fasting diets, as the name implies, is that you have to fast. Fasting feels awful, especially when we are surrounded by other people having regular eating habits. It also puts some social spotlight on your diet – explaining to your co-workers or your extended family why you are not eating on certain days is bound to generate incredulity and challenges to your diet regime.

Furthermore, even though fasting has numerous associated benefits, there are some downsides too. Fasting is associated with muscle loss, as the body doesn't discriminate between muscle mass and fat tissue when choosing cells to burn for energy.

Fasting also risks malnutrition, only by not eating enough foods to get essential nutrients. This risk can be somewhat alleviated by taking vitamin supplements and eating nutrient-rich foods, but fasting can also slow and halt the digestive system altogether – preventing the absorption of supplements. These supplements also need dietary fat to be dissolved, which you might also lack if you were to implement a strict fasting method.

On top of this, fasting isn't appropriate for a vast range of people. You don't want children to fast and potentially inhibit their growth. Likewise, the elderly, the ill, and the pregnant are all too vulnerable to the risks of fasting.

Additionally, there are several psychological detriments to fasting, despite commonly being associated with spiritual revelations. Fasting makes you irritable and causes you to feel slightly on edge – your body is telling you always that you need to forage for food, enacting physical processes that affect your mood and emotions.

This is why the authors of the Sirtfood diet sought a replacement for fasting diets. Fasting is beneficial for our body, but it just isn't practical for society at large. This is where sirtuin activators and Sirtfoods come to the rescue.

Sirtuins were first discovered in 1984 in yeast molecules. Of course, once it became apparent that sirtuin activators affected a variety of factors, such as lifespan and metabolic activity, interest in these proteins blossomed.

Sirtuin activators boost your mitochondria's activity, the part of the biological cell responsible for the production of energy. This, in turn, mirrors the energy-boosting effects, which also occur due to exercise and fasting. The Sirt food diet is thought to start a process called adipogenesis, which prevents fat cells from duplicating – which should interest any potential dieter.

The exciting part is that sirtuin activators influence your genetics. The notion of the 'genetic' lottery is embedded in the public consciousness, but genes are more changeable then you might think. You won't be able to change your eye color or height, but you can activate or deactivate specific genes based on environmental factors. This is called epigenetics, and it is a fascinating field of study.

Sirtuin activators cause the S.I.R. genes to activate, the before-mentioned 'skinny genes,' which in turn increases the release of sirtuins. Sirts or Silent Information Regulators also help regulate the circadian rhythm, which is your natural body clock and influences sleep patterns.

Sleep is essential for many vital biological processes, including those that help regulate blood sugar (which is also essential for losing weight). If you find yourself always stuck in a state of lag and brain fog, this may be caused by your circadian rhythm is out of sync, which is another way the sirtfood diet can help your body.

Additionally, sirts help contains free radicals. Free radicals are not as impressive as the sound – they are A.W.O.L. particles in your body that damage your D.N.A. and speed up the aging process.

To summarize, the Sirtfood diet contains foods which are high in sirtuin activators. Sirtuin activators activate your S.I.R. genes, or 'skinny genes,' which enact beneficial metabolic processes. These processes, which involve molecules, called Sirts, cause your body to burn fat, repair human cells, and combat free radicals.

Evidence

So, sirt foods have been hailed as the next dietary wonder – but where is the cold, hard evidence? Well, the proof of the sirt food diet comes from multiple sources. To start with, Aidan Goggins and Glen Matten, the originators of the Sirtfood diet, performed their trial at a privately-owned fitness center to test sirt foods themselves.

At a fitness center called K.X., in Chelsea, London, the two authors of the sirt food diet made a selection of their clientele eat a carefully monitored constructed sirt food diet. What is particularly interesting about the study is that weight wasn't the only variable measured – the researchers also measured body composition and metabolic activity – they were searching for the holistic effect of the diet.

97.5% of people managed to stick to the first-three day fasting period, involving only 1000 calories. Generally speaking, this is a much higher rate of success than typical fasting diets, where many people have their willpower shattered in just the first few days.

Out of the 40 participants, 39 completed the study. In terms of overall fitness and weight, the individuals in the study were well distributed – 2 were officially obese, 15 fell into the overweight category while 22 had a natural body mass index. There were also 21 women and 18 men – a diet for both the genders! However, with that being said, being members of a fitness center, the individuals in the study were more likely to exercise more than the standard population – a potential confounding factor.

Participants lost over 7lbs on average in the first week. Every participant experienced an improvement in body composition, even if their gains were not as dramatic as their peers.

There were also numerous reported psychological benefits, although these were not formally quantified.

These improvements include an overall sense of feeling and looking better. As a side note, it was also claimed the 40 participants rarely felt hungry, despite the calorie deficits imposed by the diet.

The most startling result from the sirt food diet is that muscle mass after the 1-week diet period was either the same as before, or showed slight improvements. Dieting law typically states that when losing fat, muscle is also lost, usually around 20-30% of the total weight loss, you should lose 2-3 lbs of muscle for every 10 pounds lost.

Of course, retaining muscle isn't just better from an overall fitness perspective, but also a beautiful view. A common fear, especially in men, is that if they lose weight, they will look skinny, scrawny, and unhealthy. Yet by retaining the muscle, you will gain that toned, slither look that is so fashionable in models.

Another essential reason why retaining muscle mass is your resting energy expenditure. Your muscles require energy, even when you are not using them intensely. Owing to this, people who keep skeletal muscles burn more calories than people who don't, also if both are sedentary. Being muscular allows you to eat more calories and get away with it!

Muscle mass has also been associated with a general decrease in degenerative diseases as you age (such as diabetes and osteoporosis) as well as lower rates of mental health problems (such as depression and excessive anger).

Overall, the clinical trial performed at the K.X. Fitness center not only supported the notion that the Sirtfood diet can aid weight loss and promote holistic body health, but it also leads to the surprising finding that sirt foods can retain muscle mass.

Blue Zones

The other evidence for the power of Sirtfoods comes from the 'blue zones.' The blue zones are small regions in the world where people miraculously live longer than everywhere else.

Perhaps most startlingly, you don't just see people live longer in blue zones; you still see them retain energy, vigor, and overall health even in their advanced years. Most of us have a fear of becoming decrepit, immobile, and overall miserable as we age.

Furthermore, we envision this as starting to occur in our forties and fifties, while becoming a fixed reality in our sixties, seventies, and eighties. Yet, in the blue zones, people not only live past 100 surprisingly, but can walk, work, and exercise just as well as in the younger years. Likewise, they remain mentally slither and don't suffer the cognitive deficits we typically associate with old age.

The blue zones include several areas of the Mediterranean, Japan, Italy, and Costa Rica. What do these regions all have in common? They all eat a diet high in sirt foods. The Mediterranean is famous for its healthy diet involving copious amounts of fish and olive oil. The Japanese savor matcha green tea, while the Costa Ricans traditionally indulge in cocoa, coffee, and more.

This is the beauty of the sirt food diet – it isn't trying to make your eating habits artificial and awkward. It is merely copying the healthiest practices that already exist around the world.

Chapter 20: Hacking the Skinny Gene

Taking Foods in the Plan That Are Nutritious

Acute calorie restriction just 1,000 calories daily for the phase one stage "first three days" and 1,500 daily for the rest of the week. And most of those calories should be obtained from the juice.

As you already know, restricting calories is the most dependable strategy for shedding weight. And for it is worthy, research from Finland's Helsinki University discovered that low-calorie foods might naturally improve sirtuin reaction, irrespective of whether you eat foods rich in sirtuin or not. Hence, include some few sirtuin foods to your diet: kale, walnuts, buckwheat, celery, are all great food. However, do not conclude that you cannot eat anything else. If you're determined about shedding weight, pay attention to lean protein, vegetables, and whole grains to reduce your total energy down.

You can discover your normal weight-loss calorie objective by locating your resting metabolic rate and then multiplying it by 1.3; let assume using exercise physiology and also sports nutritionist tips. Anything lesser than that, and you risk reducing your metabolism down.

Diet to Activate Sirtuins and Promote Health

It's apparently no accident that some of the individuals with long lifespan and healthiest populations in the world eat diets that are rich in these sirtuin-activating foods, examples are those in the Mediterranean and parts of Asia. The Mediterranean diet includes polyphenol-rich fruits, veggies, olive oil, including red wine. The Asian diet is rich in isoflavones present in soya beans and epigallactins from green tea.

Acquiring several of these health developing foods into your diet is proportionately easy. They can be included in many diets and even compound to make super-sirt meals!

Below are some great ideas you can get started with

Make use of olive oil for frying or roasting veggies or vegetables and salad dressings.

Ensure to own a jar of olives handy to snack on and include olives to salads or cooked meals. Tapenade usually makes a great topping for rye pieces of bread.

Exchange usual tea and coffee for green tea. Include a press of lemon for extra interest.

Miso alternatively can be used rather than stock cubes to flavor soups and stews. Milder light-colored miso may be used as a spread. Miso soup makes a great snack or soft meal if presented with salad or bread.

Include tofu or tempeh to stir-fries. Mix silken tofu into soups, immerse, and creamy desserts.

Put berries, blackcurrants to muesli, smoothies, and juices. Fresh yogurt, as well as fresh berries, ensure a healthy snack or dessert.

Take your greens. Cabbage and broccoli are outstanding support to any meal and can also be included in stir-fries, curries, stews, and casseroles.

Enrich up your life with turmeric and other spices. Don't restrict your input of seasonings to curries, include them to grains and vegetables.

Include cacao powder to smoothies and desserts too. Dredge cacao nibs on salads or include to trail mixes.

Apples are the ideal handy snack. Make sure you have one with you most times.

Buckwheat macaroni can be made as a tasty gluten complimentary option to wheat pasta, and buckwheat flour can also be made in baked products or to stiffer sauces. Buckwheat is also a great alternative that goes well with salads combined with roasted vegetables and toasted nuts.

Pros and Cons of Sirt food Diet

Pros:

- The 'sirt foods' apparently trigger the sirtuin in your body that is a type of protein that helps shield your cells from dying and contracting diseases, and also controlling your body metabolism.

- It's established on a research of 40 gym participants who each of them lost, on average 7lb in a week without losing muscle weight.

- You can eat normal amounts of dark chocolate and wine on a steady basis without you being affected.

- It consists of foods that are largely healthy and nourishing, such as blueberries, walnuts, and green tea.

- It is made to be effective for the long term and makes you healthy for life while also reducing the aging process.

Cons:

- For the first week, there is a calorie reduction that will eventually make most people lose weight, irrespective of what food is taken. This might occur as a result of the calorie restriction itself, which makes the participants shed weight. Also, for the first three days, you only take 1,000 calories daily, and the next four days requires to take up to 1,500 calories per day.

- Intensively reducing your calorie intake can be harmful if your body is not used to it and can make you sluggish.

- There is not enough proof that it follows through on its promises, most importantly the aspect of speeding up of your metabolism. Research on 40 people isn't much enough to say that it will eventually work as a healthy means to shed weight.

- You can only include foods on the sirt food list examples are 'sirt juices,' soy, green tea, and walnuts.

In the conclusion of the above, there's less significance in having a variety of foods in your diet so as to look and feel good. For instance, eating fruit and vegetable every day provides enough minerals and vitamins in your meals at all times.

Chapter 21: Exercises and Daily Commitments

The commitment to exercise regularly may appear incompatible with the rhythms and lifestyle habits of many people. It is not easy to cut time, but with stubbornness, it is possible to succeed. It is important to play sports to dispose of what we eat.

Surely the first step is to become aware of the importance of the physical activity. A more detailed handbook could help us choose the most suitable solution for our needs.

If you have time available early in the morning before breakfast or in the evening before dinner, a nice ride would be ideal. Before training, it is a good habit to have a cup of matcha tea, which increases thermogenesis, which allows the consumption of more energy.

For those who have little time but goodwill with small daily tricks, they will almost unwittingly do their physical activity. If we really cannot avoid using the car, we try to park it far from the place where we have to go, in order to walk at least 5 minutes. If we use public transport, we can get off one or two stops earlier. If we live on the penthouse, we use our foot. Going on foot is a good habit to acquire, instead of hitchhiking the car to get around.

For those who have a lot of time but little will, a method that can help overcome laziness could be to be followed by a personal trainer. Or do physical activity with more motivated friends. Having a dog can also be a great incentive to go for a walk.

Doing exercises with the help of a web tutorial, doing yoga, fitness or CrossFit are all training programs designed for those who do not have time to go to the gym and want to take some time to start exercising again.

The most difficult cases are those of those who have little time and little will. These are the cases that, like all difficult ones, should be seen as a challenge. It is appropriate to make a bet on ourselves. Maybe by proposing to try to do physical activity for a limited period, because we know habits need to be changed slowly, especially the more deeply rooted ones.

If you change your mentality, you change your physique. The greatest gratification will come when only for one's own merit will it be to be fit, full of energy and planning. Losing weight means taking care of yourself and returning to feeling good, waking up with a smile, and being energetic all day. It's just a matter of desire, time, mind, and organization.

So, we find the exercise that best suits our abilities and needs, and we try to do it regularly and consistently.

Eliminate Excess Fat

Those who follow the sirt diet should also perform physical activity. This is valid for everybody. The movement stimulates the activation of sirtuins for the benefit of health. Moreover, being overweight increases the risk of contracting serious illnesses.

Obesity, both for young people and for adults is one of the most important diseases of western society. It is associated with cardiovascular diseases, heart attack, stroke, hypertension, type 2 diabetes and debilitating diseases such as osteoarthritis, gout, and metabolic syndrome.

The most logical solution to burn excess fat is possible only if you adopt a balanced low-calorie diet, accompanied by a good level of exercise.

A non-low-calorie and balanced diet in sirt nutrients allow you to eliminate fat mass more and more, only if the diet is associated with an adequate sports program; on the contrary, the muscles will suffer.

Obviously, constancy and regularity are needed to obtain benefits from physical activity. Three hours of concentrated Sunday activities are less effective than those that will be spread over several days of the week. Then, another factor not to be underestimated is to opt for physical activities that provide some satisfaction. Our exercise must be fun, maybe even varied, to induce those who are easily bored to avoid stress.

Tone the Lean Mass

It is wrong to focus only on aerobic exercises, leaving out the anaerobic aspect and toning. Spending many hours on a treadmill certainly promotes fat consumption.

However, the excess of excessive fat loss predisposes our body to the release of the stress hormone, cortisol. It slows down the metabolism, accelerates water retention, and the perception of the feeling of general tiredness. In fact, one feels very tired and the body will be less toned.

A correct training card must take into account the basic muscle composition, for women in particular, of the targeted training needs for legs, buttocks, and abdominals, to ensure good toning for a pleasant aesthetic.

At the level of muscle growth, men and women share the same structure; the obvious difference lies in the production of natural testosterone, which obviously is higher in men and allows them to increase mass in a much more considerable way.

To obtain the desired results, therefore, we must integrate training with exercises that use weights and machines. Strength training, with weights, barbells and kettlebells, studied on individual needs, is the right way to tone your muscles.

Power-ups with tools are important for developing lean mass over fat. The calorie expenditure associated with tonic muscles is higher than the fat mass. It is possible to eat the same, following a sirt diet but consuming more calories per day. Muscle development and endurance allow bones to remain compact, useful for preventing osteoporosis.

Targeted Exercises

Training in the wrong way has, as a first effect, the failure to achieve the goal we have set. If we want to make our bodies more harmonious, toned, and lean, and we don't expect the right rules, we probably won't see the change we want.

A wrong load, excessive training intensity, a concentrated effort on some limbs or muscles increases the chances of obtaining microtraumas or other injuries. Training will soon become a source of stress and frustration, if we do not take note of our mistakes, with the only result of letting us abandon our program.

It is easy to get caught up in enthusiasm and choose to train to start from easy exercises setting your own goals, which are, of course, subjective and personal.

Aerobic activities stimulate the body to use large quantities of oxygen and help the muscles and encourage the consumption of calories.

For women who aspire to have a harmonious body and want to tone their body, it would be advisable to practice a complete workout, even at the time of music, which includes push-ups, bends, stretches, and exercises with small dumbbells and kettlebells.

Various Exercises

To work completely on the whole musculature, with harmonious effects on an aesthetic level and health benefits, a weekly training session for women must take into account the variability of the weights and the intensity of the training. Contrary to what many women think, it will not be some exercise commensurate with their body to disfigure the female body with man exercises. In any case, weight training is essential, alternating with aerobics. The equipment will be suitable for those who use them are beginners or habitual to these practices.

Below is an example of a program that requires continuous work in order to burn the largest number of energies. Obviously, it is enough to choose only one activity per session.

- Treadmill for cardio exercise - 10 minutes
- Oblique crunch for abs - 3 sets x 12 reps per side
- Crunch on the flat bench for abs - 3 sets x 15 reps
- Pelvis twists - 3 sets x max repetitions in 1 minute
- Adductor machine for inner thigh - 3 sets x 15 reps
- Abductor machine for external thigh - 3 sets x 15 reps
- Leg press for legs - 3 sets x 12 reps
- Step for cardio exercise - 15 minutes
- Elliptical trainer for cardio exercise - 10 minutes
- Presses on an inclined bench for the chest - 3 sets for 15 repetitions

- Triceps with a dumbbell behind - 3 sets for 12 reps
- Lat machine ahead for the backbones - 3 sets for 12 reps
- Exercise bike for cardio exercise - 5 minutes
- Program why you want to work on gaining muscle mass, using bodybuilding machines. You can start using light loads.
- Treadmill or stepper or elliptical - 10 minutes
- Abdominal machine for the abdominals - 25 kg of weight for 2 sets and 10 reps (to be increased up to 35 kg of weight for 3 sets with 15 reps)
- Abdominal crunch - 2 sets for 12 reps
- Leg press for legs - 40 kg weight for 2 sets and 10 reps (to be increased up to 55 kg for 3 sets and 12 reps)
- Gluteus machine for the buttocks - 10 kg of weight for 2 sets and 10 reps (to be increased up to 25 kg for 3 sets and 15 reps)
- Adductor machine for inner thigh - 15 kg of weight for 2 sets and 12 reps (to be increased up to 55 kg for 3 sets and 15 reps)
- Shoulder press for shoulders - 10 kg of weight for 2 sets and 10 reps (to be increased up to 15 kg for 3 sets and 12 reps)

- Triceps at the top cables - 10 kg weight for 2 sets and 10 repetitions (to be increased up to 20 kg for 3 sets and 12 repetitions)

- Chest press for the chest - 10 kg of weight for 2 sets and 10 reps (to be increased up to 25 kg for 3 sets and 15 reps)

- Back pulley - 10 kg weight for 2 sets and 10 reps (to be increased up to 15 kg for 3 sets and 15 reps)

- Treadmill - 5 minutes.

This training of about 3 sessions per week will be ideal if the training is carried out in a constant and gradual way.

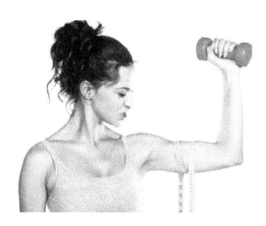

Chapter 22: 5 Truths in Sirtfood Diet

5 Truths Practically Everybody Makes Sirt Food Diet

1. Eating Foods That You Can Not Actually Like

In case You believe you are going to turn into a fan of Brussels sprouts as it's January second and you've not eaten anything in 3 months weeks, you are setting yourself up to fail. "One explanation diets do not work is they induce people to eat things that they don't really like. "If the carrot smoothie isn't exercising for you, take to sautéed lettuce, celery, tofu chips, or even better, ditch the carrot and attempt lettuce, collard greens, Swiss chard, or still another vegetable" The following secret to eating healthy without quitting life would be really to test out spices. "Do not forget to take to various seasonings or manners of cooking. By way of instance, get a Cajun spice combination or five-spice and scatter it together with one's poultry or veggies.

2. Expecting Immediate Results

The Observing you did on Christmas isn't going to become reversed following weekly --or possibly per couple to having the sh*t together (i.e., healthy eating). "The most straightforward way to fall short of one's resolution or goal is to help it become unattainable., lead nourishment specialist at Seattle Sutton's Healthy

Eating. "For example, resolving to prevent eat your favorite take-out food or planning to lose 10 lbs within 1 month may backfire. That is not because allowing the foods that you like results in finally bingeing to them once you cannot tolerate the craving. And seeking to reduce a lot of weight too fast will undoubtedly cause disappointment and also a dip bag of Doritos.

The Key would be to put smaller goals that buildup to an objective, he states. This means that you may attempt to prevent this take out joint more frequently than you can today or wish to lose a couple of pounds weekly --and soon you finally reach your target, " she states.

3. Maybe not Getting Meals in Front of Time

One of the reasons why people overeat around Christmas is there is a large amount of food outside; it is easy to catch. Whenever the Observing is finished, make it simple to choose healthful options by organizing healthy food beforehand. Like that, it is possible to arrive at it when you are hungry, rather than earning a game-time decision when you are mesmerized. "Meal preparation is critical to eating a balanced diet program. "Cut vegetables up and also make additional portions of dinner to the week beforehand. In this manner, it is possible to collect dinner to a busy week very quickly."

Now you won't think some of the strangest things a few individuals did to eliminate weight:

4. Maybe not Assessing Labels at the Supermarket

Being A little more particular regarding the foods that you buy at the store will be able to assist you in getting right back on the right track after ingestion that which without any difficulty. Examine the food labels to the ingredients you have to produce a more informed decision regarding whether it belongs in what you eat plan. Chen says it especially crucial to pay careful attention to serving sizes. "A jar of juice might actually comprise two portions," she states. This means it includes twice the calories and sugar just as what's recorded on the tag. And as you are not likely in the habit of just drinking half a juice, then which will prevent you from losing weight," says Chen. Other critical elements to consider will be the total amount of protein and fiber in meals. Take ¼ tsp of fiber and 4 tsp of protein into every Meal to remain full and fulfilled.

5. Maybe not Acquiring a Backup Policy for Seconds Weakness

Putting A strategy set up to modify your daily diet is fantastic. However, you've also must policy for roadblocks. Simply take stress eating throughout an especially annoying afternoon, such as. Once you learn, you are enticed to make yourself feel a lot better with the assistance of ice cream, then look for a backup program. Maybe you opt to find yourself a 20-minute massage at a nail salon or blow some steam off from the particular candlelight yoga class. "Both are welcome adjustments to a healthier new way of life, and you'll feel far better in the long term."

Conclusion

When we cut back on calories, it makes a deficiency of energy that activates what is known as the "skinny gene." This triggers a raft of positive changes. It places the body into a sort of endurance mode where it quits putting away fat and normal development forms are required to be postponed. Rather, the body directs its concentration toward consuming its stores of fat and turning on ground-breaking housekeeping qualities that repair and rejuvenate our cells, adequately giving them a spring cleaning. The result is weight loss and improved protection from sickness.

In any case, the same number of health food nuts know, cutting calories includes some major disadvantages. Temporarily, the decrease in energy consumption incites hunger, touchiness, exhaustion, and muscle loss. Longer-term calorie limitation makes our digestion deteriorate. This is the destruction of all calorie-prohibitive diets and makes ready for the weight to return heaping on. It is thus that 99 percent of weight watchers are destined to flop over the long run.

The entirety of this drove us to pose a major inquiry: is it somehow possible to activate our thin quality with all the extraordinary advantages that brings without expecting to stick to serious calorie limitation with every one of those downsides?

Enter Sirtfoods, a newfound group of wonder nourishments. Sirtfoods are especially wealthy in exceptional supplements that, when we consume them, can initiate skinny qualities in our bodies that calorie limitation does. These qualities are known as sirtuins. They originally became exposed in a milestone concentrate in 2003 when specialists found that resveratrol, a compound found in red grape skin and red wine, significantly expanded the life expectancy of yeast. Incredibly, resveratrol had a similar impact on life span as calorie limitation, yet this was accomplished without reducing energy consumption. Beginning time considers show resveratrol ensures against the antagonistic impacts of fatty, high-fat, and high-sugar counts calories; advances healthy maturing by deferring age-related infections; and increments fitness. it has been appeared to impersonate the impacts of calorie limitation and exercise.

With the discovery of resveratrol, the universe of health research was on the cusp of something important, and the pharmaceutical business industry wasted no time committing. Scientists started screening a large number of various synthetic substances for their capacity to enact our sirtuin qualities. This uncovered various characteristic plant mixes, not only resveratrol, with critical sirtuin-actuating properties. It was additionally found that a given food could contain an entire range of these plant mixes, which could work in show to both guide retention and amplify that food's sirtuin-enacting impact. This had been one of the huge puzzles around resveratrol. The researchers exploring different avenues regarding resveratrol regularly expected to use far higher portions than we know give an advantage when devoured as a feature of red wine. However, just as resveratrol, red wine contains a variety of other normal plant mixes, including high measures of piceatannol just as quercetin, myricetin, and epicatechin, every one of which was appeared to autonomously enact our sirtuin qualities and, progressively significant, to work in coordination.

The issue for the pharmaceutical business is that they can't showcase a group of supplements or nourishments as the following large blockbuster drug. So, all things being equal they contributed a huge number of dollars to create and direct preliminaries of manufactured mixes with expectations of revealing a Shangri-La pill. At present various investigations of sirtuin-initiating drugs are in progress for a large number of interminable illnesses, just as the first-historically speaking FDA-affirmed preliminary to explore whether a medication can slow maturing.

As tempting as that may appear, if history has shown us anything, it's that we ought not to hold out a lot of trust in this pharmaceutical ambrosia. Over and over the pharmaceutical and health businesses have attempted to imitate the advantages of nourishments and diets through disengaged medications and supplements. What's more, consistently it's missed the mark. Why hang tight ten or more years for the authorizing of these supposed miracle drugs, and the unavoidable symptoms they bring, when right now we have all the amazing advantages accessible readily available through the food we eat?

So, while the pharmaceutical business constantly seeks after a drug like magic projectile, we need to retrain our attention on diet.

FAQ

Is it OK to Exercise During Phase 1 of the Program?

Nothing wrong can come if you exercise during this phase of the sirt food diet. Moderate exercise is highly recommended, but if you choose to go for intense training, keep in mind that this will use up your energy reserves (most likely). If you are used to a moderate level of training, then the best way is to continue the same level during the first phase of this program. Intense exercise can do the fat burning for you, but it can also make you feed again, although you shouldn't have to. Therefore, keep it moderate and let the sirt food diet do the work for you.

What's the Purpose of Following This Diet if I'm Already Slim?

The first phase of the sirt food diet should not be tried by underweight people. How can you tell if you are underweight? Just check your body mass index (BMI) level. Any person with a BMI below 18.5 is considered underweight, so phase 1 of this program should not be tried by them. Keep in mind that the maintenance phase can also lead to fat loss, but it can help you build muscle as well. The underweight people should benefit from the activation of sirtuins, but they need to consume a lot less amount of food compared to overweight people.

Is the Sirtfood Diet Right For Me if I'm Obese?

Although a small number of participants in the pilot study were obese, I can only encourage obese people to try this diet in the long term. Why? Because it creates the perfect environment in your body to lose weight. Obese people need to lose weight constantly in the long run, not to lose a lot of weight dramatically in a very short amount of time. If this diet worked for people and they lost seven pounds in seven days, this rate could be considered satisfactory for them. However, they need to alternate the first phase and the second phase.

I Managed to Reach the Weight I Want, and I Simply Don't Want to Lose Any More Weight. Do I have to Stop Eating sirt Foods?

Achieving your objectives can only prove that this diet works. So, the first phase worked like a charm for you. Even though you don't want to lose any more weight, you can stick to the maintenance phase for a long time. You have to benefit from sirtuins for life. After all, this diet is also about health benefits, and if you have a good thing running, why stop it? You can choose your ingredients wisely to avoid weight loss and gain muscle mass, as the sirt food diet can allow you this option as well.

I've Just Finished Phase 2. Do I Need to Stop Drinking the Green Juice?

Short answer: no. You can still have your morning green juice, as this powerful morning cocktail is the magic potion that can boost the productivity of the sirtuin-activating nutrients. If you want to benefit from the consumption of sirt foods, you should never stop drinking the morning green juice.

Is it OK to Follow This Diet if I Take Medication?

The sirt food diet can be tried by mostly everyone, but there are a few exceptions. When you are sick and on medication, nutrient deprivation is not something that you need, plus the sirt food diet can mess with the medication you are taking.

Can Children Try This Diet?

The sirt food diet was designed to be enjoyed by most of the family, including children. If you have the chance to keep your children away from junk food, why shouldn't you let them reap the benefits of sirt foods? Obviously, you don't want your children to be hooked on coffee and green tea, and obviously not on red wine. But most of the other ingredients can be tried by children.

CPSIA information can be obtained
at www.ICGtesting.com
Printed in the USA
BVHW091503150221
600147BV00006B/494